M(odified) E(ssay) Q(uestions) for Medicine Finals

With Solutions and Tips

Volume 3

Other World Scientific Titles by the Editor

M(odified) E(ssay) Q(uestions) for Medicine Finals
With Solutions and Tips
Volume 2
ISBN: 978-981-3109-54-4
ISBN: 978-981-3109-55-1 (pbk)

M(odified) E(ssay) Q(uestions) for Medicine Finals
With Solutions and Tips
ISBN: 978-981-4412-28-5 (pbk)

M(odified) E(ssay) Q(uestions) for Medicine Finals

With Solutions and Tips

Volume 3

editors

Derrick Chen Wee Aw
C. Rajasoorya

Sengkang General Hospital, Singapore

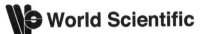
World Scientific

NEW JERSEY · LONDON · SINGAPORE · BEIJING · SHANGHAI · HONG KONG · TAIPEI · CHENNAI · TOKYO

Published by

World Scientific Publishing Co. Pte. Ltd.

5 Toh Tuck Link, Singapore 596224

USA office: 27 Warren Street, Suite 401-402, Hackensack, NJ 07601

UK office: 57 Shelton Street, Covent Garden, London WC2H 9HE

British Library Cataloguing-in-Publication Data
A catalogue record for this book is available from the British Library.

M(ODIFIED) E(SSAY) Q(UESTIONS) FOR MEDICINE FINALS
With Solutions and Tips
Volume 3

ISBN 978-981-122-855-1 (hardcover)
ISBN 978-981-123-009-7 (paperback)
ISBN 978-981-122-856-8 (ebook for institutions)
ISBN 978-981-122-857-5 (ebook for individuals)

For any available supplementary material, please visit
https://www.worldscientific.com/worldscibooks/10.1142/12049#t=suppl

Contents

Foreword   ix
Preface   xi
List of Contributors   xiii

Assessment Paper 1   **1**

Question 1.1   2
Question 1.2   5
Question 1.3   10
Question 1.4   16
Question 1.5   20

Assessment Paper 2   **27**

Question 2.1   28
Question 2.2   32
Question 2.3   36
Question 2.4   40
Question 2.5   43

Assessment Paper 3   **47**

Question 3.1   48
Question 3.2   52
Question 3.3   56
Question 3.4   61
Question 3.5   66

Assessment Paper 4   **69**

Question 4.1   70

Question 4.2   74
Question 4.3   79
Question 4.4   85
Question 4.5   89

Assessment Paper 5   **93**

Question 5.1   94
Question 5.2   99
Question 5.3   102
Question 5.4   107
Question 5.5   113

Assessment Paper 6   **119**

Question 6.1   120
Question 6.2   125
Question 6.3   128
Question 6.4   133
Question 6.5   138

Assessment Paper 7   **143**

Question 7.1   144
Question 7.2   150
Question 7.3   155
Question 7.4   158
Question 7.5   164

Assessment Paper 8   **169**

Question 8.1   170
Question 8.2   173
Question 8.3   177
Question 8.4   182
Question 8.5   187

Assessment Paper 9   **191**

Question 9.1   192
Question 9.2   198
Question 9.3   202
Question 9.4   206
Question 9.5   212

Assessment Paper 10   **217**

Question 10.1   218
Question 10.2   222
Question 10.3   226
Question 10.4   230
Question 10.5   235

Solutions   **239**

Foreword

Taking a professional exam is probably one of the most stressful experiences of our lives. Having been an examiner for many years in my own specialty, I know that the candidate often wonders: "What is in the examiner's mind?"

In this book, an experienced team of examiners — well respected, practising clinicians — have penned their experiences to share with you. This is not only a valuable bank for exam preparation but also a good source of information for daily practice shared in a distilled and practical manner.

I have worked with both A/Prof Aw and Prof Raja for many years. A/Prof Aw's passion for teaching is infectious, and his dermatology books are gems indeed. Professor Raja was my mentor when I was a medical officer, and his dedication to the education of the next generation is admirable. Both are respected and esteemed clinicians and well liked as teachers and mentors. Their ability to make a complex topic simple and their passion for teaching are legendary.

I am honoured and delighted to write this foreword for the third volume of the *MEQs for Medicine Finals* series. This book builds upon the first two volumes, and the Medicine team in Sengkang General Hospital, where specialists are part of the general internal medicine practice, has contributed to this endeavour. This gives the unique opportunity for specialists to directly share their perspectives and thinking behind problems presenting in the general medicine patient. It also provides more perspectives on dealing with the complex medical patient. I am confident that this book will not only be valuable for your examination preparations but also in your daily practice.

Associate Professor Ong Biauw Chi
Chairman Medical Board, Sengkang General Hospital

I had the privilege of looking through the first volume of "Modified Essay Questions (MEQs) for Medicine Finals". The 10 papers within consisted of a treasure trove of real-life cases that were followed by probing questions. These quizzes manage to strike a balance between being "too easy" (and thus "not interesting enough") and "too exotic", and may be considered trivia by some. In fact, I think the way the case studies were structured provoke much curiosity to search beyond the questions presented. I have no doubt the same will be found in this volume, which is co-edited by the two titans of education and medicine, Prof Raja and A/Prof Derrick Aw. The practice of medicine may be evolving at an ever-faster pace, though the fundamental principles of problem-solving as they are promoted here will remain constant. The seed of lifelong learning based on enduring curiosity is found in every page of this masterpiece, which we should all treasure and behold.

Professor Christopher Cheng Wai Sum
Chief Executive Officer, Sengkang General Hospital

Preface

The materials for this edition come from a brand new team of writers — friends and colleagues at my new workplace, the Department of General Medicine in Sengkang General Hospital. In fact, I was particularly thrilled to co-edit these modified essay questions (MEQs) with Prof C Rajasoorya. He is our campus education director and is also a legend and inspiration to all of us in the field of Internal Medicine. As we endeavor to generate a high-quality examination practice with an emphasis on "application-type questions", the whole process from conception to writing, editing and vetting for *each* MEQ can take up to six hours! As per previous volumes, please try to complete each paper within 1.5 hours. A total score of 75% and above is indicative of a very good performance. As you review your answers against the recommended solutions, take time to reflect deeply and read around areas in which you have found your understanding wanting. As for readers who are already seasoned examiners, we hope that this book gives you more ideas on setting questions. Enjoy.

Derrick Aw Chen Wee

Examinations are a formidable task even for the best prepared. My role as a clinician and an examiner over the decades has made me realise that most students put in a lot of effort in preparation. However, they are not cognisant of the reasoning process involved and the thinking behind questions asked and the answers expected (perhaps this is what some call "study smart", something I was ignorant of as a medical student years ago). Of course, the questions asked are partly influenced by examiner bias — in the current context, examiners and their teams have taken efforts to minimise this bias.

Contexualisation for an individual patient within the framework of data available often guides our practice in real life, but somehow this is not exhibited during exams. We have attempted to correct this deficiency as an audacious goal in this volume. We have targeted in this volume that students learn contextualised thinking and reasoning. We use common sense, and in some instances, rarer but engaging real-life clinical scenarios to get a student to deduce, reason out, understand the hidden traps in questions asked and think of more common possibilities. What you may find very unusual in some of the questions are facts you may passively learn just from reading the questions without even knowing the answers. The success of any volume of question items is always determined by the eventual outcome, which can make a difference for the patients under our care — if the student feels interested in the pursuit of doing more questions and puts into practice what they have learnt, we believe we have headed in the right direction.

C Rajasoorya

List of Contributors

(alphabetical order)

Adeline Chuo Mee Leh
Angela Koh Fang Yung
Chris Kong San Choon
C Rajasoorya
Deanna Lee Wai Ching
Denise Tan Yan
Derrick Aw Chen Wee
Donovan Tay Yu-Kwang
Grace Yang
Jade Soh Xiao Jue
Jessica Tan Han Ying
Jonathan Ye Qinhao
Koo Wen Hsin
Laura Tay Bee Gek
Lin Cui Li
Loh Jiashen
Mayank Chawla
Melvin Chua Peng Wei
Moy Wai Lun
Naing Chaw Su
Priscilla Chiam Pei Sze
Shashidhar Baikunje
Stanley Angkodjojo
Ubaidullah Shaik Dawood
Yeoh Lee Ying

Assessment Paper

1

Question 1.1

A 90-year-old woman presented with recurrent falls for the past year. Her medical problems were hypertension, hyperlipidaemia, diabetes mellitus (on diet control) and atrial fibrillation. Her medications included losartan 50 mg OM, simvastatin 10 mg ON and aspirin 100 mg OM. She is independent in her activities of daily living and ambulates without aid.

1. **What physical assessments would you carry out to ascertain the cause of her recurrent falls?** (4 marks)

   a. ....

   b. ....

   c. ....

   d. ....

2. **Suggest two investigations that you would order to assist in the management and prevention of future falls?** (2 marks)

   a. ....

   b. ....

A week later, she presented to the emergency department with right hip pain after she had a fall. She was diagnosed with a right neck of femur fracture. She and her family were keen for an operation, which was performed the following day.

On day three of hospitalisation, the family reported that the patient appeared confused and did not recognise them. That night, she did not sleep and tried to climb out of bed, asking to go home.

3. **Identify the clinical syndrome** (1 mark)

....

4A. **What bedside diagnostic instrument could you use to confirm this?** (1 mark)

....

4B. **Which of the following features are mandatory criteria for the diagnosis? Select two.** (1 mark)

a. Acute onset
b. Flight of ideas
c. Inattention
d. Rambling speech
e. Stable course
f. Transient loss of consciousness ( ) & ( )

5. **Suggest three MOST likely causes that may have caused the development of this clinical syndrome.** (3 marks)

a. ....

b. ....

c. ....

As she kept trying to climb out of bed, she was bodily restrained. Two days later, she developed bilateral lower limb swelling. Vital signs were stable.

6.   Give three MOST likely explanations for the swelling.
                                                              (3 marks)

a. ....

b. ....

c. ....

On day seven of hospitalisation, the patient became very drowsy and less responsive.

7.   Give three MOST likely causes for this altered mental state.   (3 marks)

a. ....

b. ....

c. ....

Clinical examination revealed a new right-sided weakness. By day eight, the patient fortunately became more alert.

8.   List two aspects of patient assessment to help determine her prognosis, care goals and discharge planning.
                                                              (2 marks)

a. ....

b. ....

Question 1.2

A 79-year-old lady presented with giddiness for the past one week. She described it as "lightheadedness", which improved on resting. She noted some breathlessness on exertion but had no chest pain or diaphoresis. There was no limb weakness, numbness or ear symptoms.

Her past medical history consisted of hyperlipidaemia on simvastatin 20 mg ON, hypertension on amlodipine 10 mg OM and atenolol 50 mg ON, and diabetes on metformin 500 mg BD. She was also on aspirin 100 mg OM.

On examination, her vital signs were: blood pressure 110/85 mmHg, heart rate 50/min and oxygen saturation 98% on room air. Chest auscultation revealed a soft systolic murmur on the left sternal edge and vesicular breath sounds. Her abdomen was soft, with no organomegaly. The neurological examination was unremarkable.

1. **What insights concerning her clinical presentation can you obtain with careful examination of the peripheral pulse?** (3 marks)

    ....

    ....

    ....

2. **State four other bedside examinations or investigations that you could perform to complete your assessment of this patient's giddiness.** (4 marks)

a. ....

b. ....

c. ....

d. ....

Posteroanterior (PA) and left lateral chest x-rays were performed.

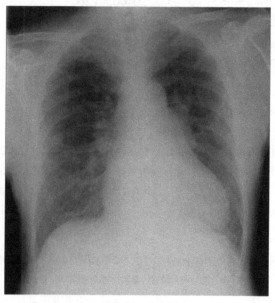

Image courtesy of Dr Uppaluri Srinivas Anandswaroop.

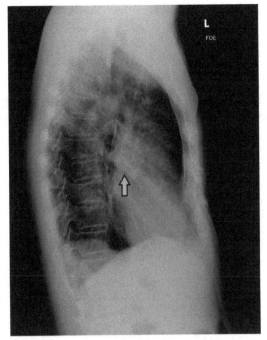

Image courtesy of Dr Uppaluri Srinivas Anandswaroop.

3A. Identify the abnormality marked with an arrow. (1 mark)

....

3B. Identify two other radiological abnormalities. (2 marks)

a. ....

b. ....

In view of her murmur, 2D echocardiography was performed:

Mild dilatation of left ventricle, EF 50%. No regional wall motion abnormality. Normal diastolic function. No pericardial effusion or thrombus. Mild calcification of mitral valve. Aortic velocity ≥4 m/s, aortic valve area ≤ 0.9 cm^2 and aortic mean gradient 40 mmHg.

4.   What is the diagnosis?   (2 marks)

....

5.   Give four potential clinical complications may arise from this condition.   (2 marks)

a. ....

b. ....

c. ....

d. ....

6.   In the light of this diagnosis, which two medications should be replaced?   (1 mark)

a. Aspirin
b. Amlodipine
c. Atenolol
d. Metformin
e. Simvastatin   (   ) & (   )

7.   Suggest two appropriate treatment interventions.
                                                (2 marks)

a. ....

b. ....

This lady declined interventions. Two months later, she was re-admitted for dark stools. Whilst she was haemodynamically stable, her haemoglobin fell from 11 to 8 g/dL.

8. **Suggest three MOST likely causes for this presentation.**

(3 marks)

a. ....

b. ....

c. ....

Question 1.3

A 40-year-old cleaner has itchy skin and rashes on and off since childhood. Whenever she gets a "flare", she consults a general practitioner who will prescribe her several topical medications that will improve the rash, but it inevitably returns with a variable degree. She now presents with one of these flares on her arms and flanks.

She has mild hypertension, for which she is taking atenolol 50 mg OM. Her weight is 55 kg, and her height is 1.70 m. She recently got married and is planning to start a family.

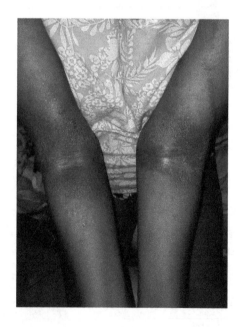

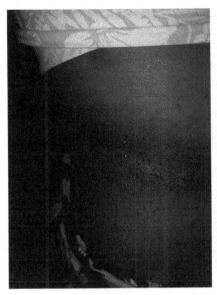 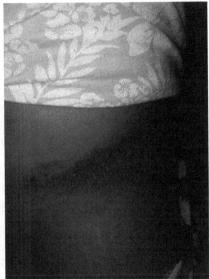

1. **Describe the morphology of the rash.** (2 marks)

....

2. **Which of the following additional site of involvement would be compatible with the clinical picture?** (1 mark)

   a. Lateral hairline
   b. Nasolabial fold
   c. Nipples
   d. Toe webspaces
   e. Umbilicus   (   )

3. **Which of the following is true in regard to the itch?**
    (2 marks)

    a. Better with antiseptic gels
    b. Better with antifungal powders
    c. Worse in early mornings
    d. Worse with cold showers
    e. Worse with sweating   (   )

4. **Which of the following concomitant dermatoses is MOST likely to be present in this patient?** (1 mark)

    a. Acne vulgaris
    b. Cysts and sinuses in groins
    c. "Dirty neck" appearance
    d. Hypertrichosis
    e. Skin tags   (   )

5. **Which of the following is the MOST appropriate topical corticosteroid formulation for this patient's dermatosis?**
    (2 marks)

    a. Cream
    b. Gel
    c. Ointment
    d. Solution
    e. Tincture   (   )

6. **Which of the following are the MOST important consid-erations for potency when selecting a topical cortico-steroid for this patient? Choose TWO.** (2 marks)

   a. The chronicity of the lesion
   b. The dimensions of the lesion
   c. The patient's preference
   d. The site of the lesion
   e. The symptomatology of the lesion
   f. The tendency to recur 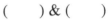 ( ) & ( )

She also complains of a painful, itchy and "wet" rash on her hands.

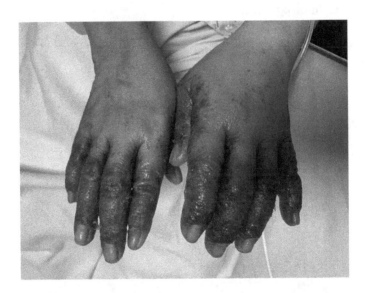

7. **What is the MOST likely diagnosis?** (2 marks)

   a. Acute cellulitis
   b. Impetigo
   c. Irritant contact dermatitis
   d. Flare of atopic dermatitis
   e. Tinea manuum ( )

8.   **Which of the following in the history would be MOST compatible with this clinical appearance?**   (2 marks)

    a. She recently dyed her hair by herself
    b. She recently "touched" a person with scabies
    c. She was away from work for two weeks
    d. She was deployed to discard used chemicals
    e. She wore silver rings on her fingers all day   (   )

9.   **Which of the following is the MOST appropriate treatment?**   (2 marks)

    a. Oral cloxacillin
    b. Parenteral glucocorticoid course
    c. Potassium permanganate compresses
    d. Regular hand moisturising
    e. Superpotent topical corticosteroid   (   )

The patient defaulted on her follow-up after receiving treatment. Half a year later, she re-presented with a flare on her trunk and limbs.

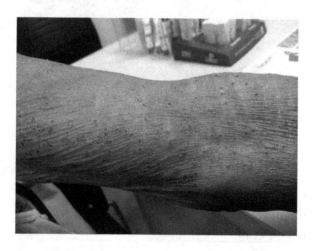

10. What is the MOST likely diagnosis?   (2 marks)

   a. Acute bacterial folliculitis
   b. Eczema herpeticum
   c. Erythema multiforme
   d. Flare of atopic eczema
   e. Pustular psoriasis   (   )

11. Which of the following is the MOST appropriate treatment?   (1 mark)

   a. Intramuscular triamcinolone
   b. Intravenous vancomycin
   c. Oral aciclovir
   d. Oral cephalexin
   e. Oral prednisolone   (   )

In view of the longstanding nature of her condition and the recurrent episodes of skin flares, the doctor discussed long-term systemic therapeutic options with her.

12. Which of the following is the MOST appropriate systemic treatment for her?   (1 mark)

   a. Azathioprine
   b. Ciclosporin
   c. Methotrexate
   d. Phototherapy
   e. Prednisolone   (   )

Question 1.4

A 56-year-old lady with a 5-year history of Type 2 diabetes mellitus presented to the emergency department with lethargy, abdominal discomfort and dyspnoea for four days. She also had multiple vomiting episodes daily. Her regular medications were metformin 1 g BD, sitagliptin 100 mg OM and gliclazide MR 30 mg OM. Due to her poor oral intake, she had suspended all her oral diabetes medications for the past three days.

Her capillary blood glucose read 23.9 mmol/L and her basic bio-chemistry revealed the following:

Urea	8.3 mmol/L	(2.7–6.9)
Sodium	135 mmol/L	(136–146)
Potassium	3.9 mmol/L	(3.5–5.1)
Chloride	106 mmol/L	(98–107)
Bicarbonate	20 mmol/L	(19–29)
Glucose	25.7 mmol/L	(3.9–11.0)
Creatinine	54 μmol/L	(45–84)
Serum Ketones	3.9 mmol/L	(0.0–0.6)

The arterial blood gas showed:

pH	7.168	(7.35–7.45)
pCO_2	17.4 mmHg	(35–45)
pO_2	99.3 mmHg	(75–100)
Standard Bicarbonate	19 mmol/L	(21–27)

1. **What is the MOST likely clinical syndrome? Justify.**

(3 marks)

....

....

2. **Comment on and explain the serum bicarbonate level in the context of this clinical syndrome.** (2 marks)

....

....

3. **Which of the following pathogenic pathways are likely to be occurring in this patient? Select three.** (3 marks)

   a. Increase in gluconeogenesis
   b. Increase in glucose utilisation by peripheral tissues
   c. Increase in glycogenesis
   d. Increase in ketones clearance
   e. Increase in level of counter-regulatory hormones
   f. Reduction in effective insulin concentration
   g. Reduction in glycogenolysis
   h. Reduction in hepatic fatty acid oxidation
   i. Reduction in level of pro-inflammatory cytokines
   j. Transient insulin sensitivity   ( ), ( ), ( )

The patient was started on aggressive intravenous hydration and continuous intravenous insulin infusion.

4.   **How often should the capillary blood glucose be checked while the patient is on insulin infusion? Explain why.**

(2 marks)

....

5A.   **How will you manage the hypokalaemia? Explain your answer.**

(2 marks)

....

....

5B.   **How often should serum potassium be checked while the patient is on insulin infusion?**

(1 mark)

....

With these measures, the patient's clinical syndrome resolves, and you would like to convert her from intravenous to subcutaneous insulin, beginning with an overlap period.

6.   **Why is it important to overlap the intravenous and subcutaneous insulin during the conversion?**

(2 marks)

....

....

The patient reports that her meal times are erratic and she sometimes skips meals.

7. **Suggest the MOST appropriate insulin regime for her. Justify.** (2 marks)

....

....

8A. **List four "danger symptoms" you would warn patients of when starting on subcutaneous insulin.** (2 marks)

a. ....

b. ....

c. ....

d. ....

8B. **Suggest an immediate action she can take at home if she experiences a "danger symptom".** (1 mark)

....

Question 1.5

A 46-year-old lady with a background of obesity, type 2 diabetes, fatty liver and epilepsy presented with seizures on awakening in the morning. She had a fever and non-bilious vomiting of two days' duration. The seizures aborted in the emergency department with intravenous lorazepam. She was admitted to the high dependency unit due to a low Glasgow Coma Scale (GCS) of 3/15 and hypotension. She remained tachycardic and hypotensive in spite of a fluid challenge. On examination, her pupils were 5 mm and reactive. Plantar reflexes were equivocal. There were no other focal neurological signs. The rest of the examination was unremarkable.

Multiple investigations were performed.

Haemoglobin	14.5 g/dL	(12–16)
WBC Count	16.47 × 10(9)/L	(4–10)
Platelet Count	467 × 10(9)/L	(140–440)
Blood Urea	2 mmol/L	(2.7–6.9)
Sodium	126 mmol/L	(136–146)
Potassium	3.2 mmol/L	(3.5–5.1)
Bicarbonate	14.8 mmol/L	(19–29)
Chloride	93 mmol/L	(98–107)
Serum Creatinine	118 μmol/L	(45–84)
Lactate	10 mmol/L	(0.5–2.2)
Creatinine Kinase	10233 U/L	(44–201)
Carbamazepine Level	3.0 mg/L	(4–12)

CRP	0.6 mg/L	(0.2–9.1)
Serum Procalcitonin	2.97 mcg/L	(<0.49)
Troponin T	314 ng/L	(<= 19)

ECG sinus tachycardia
Chest x-ray unremarkable.

1. What was the primary reason for performing a chest X-ray at the emergency department? (1 mark)

   a. Look for aspiration pneumonia
   b. Look for community-acquired pneumonia
   c. Look for fluid overload
   d. Look for lung cancer
   e. Look for pulmonary tuberculosis   ( )

2. Identify three MOST likely precipitants of her seizures. (3 marks)

   a. ....

   b. ....

   c. ....

3. Which of the following is the MOST likely explanation for the raised troponin T level? (1 mark)

   a. Acute myocardial infarction
   b. End-stage renal disease
   c. Pericarditis/myocarditis
   d. Pulmonary embolism
   e. Sequela of generalised tonic-clonic seizures   ( )

4.   Which of the following measures is the MOST important to prevent worsening of her kidney function at this stage?   (2 marks)

   a. Aggressive hydration
   b. Continuous haemofiltration
   c. Emergency haemodialysis
   d. Urgent sodium replacement
   e. Urinary alkalinisation   (   )

In spite of medical intervention, her urine output remained poor. Her blood pressure was maintained with dual inotropic support.
   Repeat and additional blood results were performed.

Hb	11.9 g/dl	(12–16)
WBC Count	5.87 × 10(9)	(4–10)
Platelet	76 × 10(9)	(140–440)

Blood Urea	5.6 mmol/L	(2.7–6.9)
Potassium	5.1 mmol/L	(3.5–5.1)
Bicarbonate	11.3 mmol/L	(19–29)
Serum Creatinine	234 µmol/L	(45–84)
Lactate	12.3 mmol/L	(0.5–2.2)
Creatine Kinase	10233 U/L	(44–201)
Corrected Calcium	1.78 mmol/L	(2.09–2.46)
Phosphate	2.78 mmol/L	(0.94–1.5)

Serum Protein	51 g/L	(68–85)
Serum Albumin	32 g/L	(40–51)
Serum Bilirubin, Total	94 umol/L	(7–32)
Serum Alkaline Phosphatase	88 U/L	(39–99)

| Serum Alanine Transaminase | 303 U/L | (6–66) |
| Serum Aspartate Transaminase | 752 U/L | (12–42) |

Urine Dipstix: positive for blood, negative for protein, leucocytes and nitrite.
UFEME: no RBCs.

5A. What diagnostic urinary test is the MOST appropriate?
(1 mark)

   a. Urinary calcium
   b. Urinary creatinine
   c. Urinary free cortisol
   d. Urinary myoglobin
   e. Urine phase contrast microscopy   (   )

5B. What diagnostic blood test is the MOST appropriate?
(1 mark)

   a. Arterial blood gas
   b. Lactate dehydrogenase
   c. Plasma cortisol
   d. Plasma myoglobin
   e. Prothombin time   (   )

6. What is the MOST appropriate management of her hypocalcaemia?
(1 mark)

   a. Check serum parathyroid hormone
   b. Enteral calcium replacement
   c. Expectant management
   d. Intravenous calcium replacement
   e. Investigate for urinary loss   (   )

7. **What is the MOST optimal renal replacement therapy for this patient?** (1 mark)

....

Her GCS remains persistently low at 4/15, and she was referred to a neurologist. The neurological assessment was unchanged. Plantar reflexes were equivocal bilaterally. However, the neurologist noticed conjunctival suffusion and subconjunctival haemorrhage. A CT brain scan showed no acute intracranial haemorrhage or large territorial infarct.

8. **Identify three MOST likely possibilities for her persistently low GCS.** (3 marks)

a. ....

b. ....

c. ....

A lumbar puncture was performed.

CSF Examination: Appearance clear
Opening Pressure: 40 cmH$_2$O, closing pressure 35 cmH$_2$O

Protein	0.95 g/L	(0.15–0.45)
RBC count	593/microL	
WBC count	95/microL	
Lymphocytes	0	
Polymorphs	97%	
Monocytes	3%	

Bacterial gram stain negative, culture negative
Meningitis multiplex-PCR negative
AFB smear/culture, TB PCR awaited

Fungal microscopy negative, culture awaited
Cytology: Inflammatory yield

Additional blood tests revealed:

HIV serology negative
Serum cryptococcal antigen negative

9A. What is your interpretation of the lumbar puncture results? (3 marks)

....

....

9B. What cerebrospinal fluid (CSF) parameter is missing, and what is its diagnostic value? (1 mark)

....

10. Suggest the MOST likely infectious agent in this patient. (1 mark)

....

On the fourth day of admission, the patient acutely desaturated and required mechanical ventilation.

11. Given your understanding of the infection, propose an explanation for the sudden deterioration. (1 mark)

....

Assessment Paper
2

Question 2.1

A 35-year-old lady at her 28-week gestation period presented to the emergency department with a complaint of worsening epigastric pain. She reported intermittent epigastric discomfort over several years that worsened last month with nausea and vomiting. She denied passing black stool or having any symptoms of overt bleeding. She is a vegan and only takes a prenatal vitamin daily.

Clinically, her heart rate was 94/min and blood pressure 180/100 mmHg. The abdominal examination was notable for a gravid uterus and mild epigastric tenderness.

Her full blood count showed the following:

Haemoglobin	8.8 g/dL	(12–16)
WBC Count	11.39 × 10(9)/L	(4–10)
Platelet Count	90 × 10(9)/L	(140–440)
MCV	75.7 fL	(78.0–98.0)
MCH	22.2 pg	(27.0–32.0)
MCHC	29.3 g/dL	(32.0–36.0)
RBC Distribution Width	16.7%	(10.9–15.7)

1A. What is the MOST important condition to be excluded at this time? (2 marks)

....

1B. **List three relevant physical signs that you would specifically look for in this patient.** (3 marks)

a. ....

b. ....

c. ....

1C. **Which of the following urgent confirmatory laboratory investigations should be performed? Check four brackets.** (0.5 × 4 = 2 marks)

a. Peripheral blood smear   ( )
b. Serum direct bilirubin   ( )
c. Serum lactic acid   ( )
d. Serum lactate dehydrogenase   ( )
e. Ultrasound hepatobiliary system   ( )
f. Ultrasound kidneys   ( )
g. Urinalysis   ( )
h. Liver function test   ( )

2. **Based on the *history* alone, suggest three MOST likely causes for her anaemia.** (3 marks)

a. ....

b. ....

c. ....

3. **Which of the following is the MOST appropriate management of her blood pressure?** (2 marks)

   a. Induction of labour
   b. Intramuscular dexamethasone
   c. Intravenous labetalol
   d. Sublingual glyceryl trinitrate
   e. Urgent Caesarean section   ( )

During hospitalisation, further studies were performed to evaluate
the anaemia:

Serum Iron	2 umol/L	(8–32)
Serum Transferrin	1.0 g/L	(2.0–3.6)
Serum Ferritin	7.2 ug/L	(13.0–150.0)
Total Iron Binding Capacity	26 umol/L	(39–60)
Transferrin Saturation	7.7%	(≤50)

4A. **Base on the laboratory values provided what type of
anaemia does this patient have?** (2 marks)

....

4B. **Which of the following is the MOST appropriate management of her anaemia?** (2 marks)

   a. High-dose oral iron replacement
   b. Intravenous iron replacement
   c. No specific treatment is necessary at this stage
   d. Transfusion of four units of platelets
   e. Transfusion of two units of packed red cells   ( )

Subsequent non-invasive testing was positive for *Helicobactor
pylori* infection, but treatment was deferred due to the lady's
pregnancy.

At three months post-partum, the lady's repeat haemoglobin was 12.2 g/dL and platelet count 115 × 10(9)/L. She brought her health screening results from two years ago, which showed a platelet count of 120 × 10(9)/L. She had just found out that she had chronic Hepatitis B during her antenatal screening.

5A. **Give two MOST likely differential diagnoses for her thrombocytopaenia.** (2 marks)

a. ....

b. ....

5B. **For each of your differential diagnosis, respectively, suggest one investigation and/or intervention to evaluate it.** (2 marks)

a. ....

b. ....

Question 2.2

A 23-year-old female presented to the emergency department with a 2-week history of intermittent fever. This was associated with headache and myalgia. She had just returned from a 3-month mission trip to Indonesia, Vietnam and New Zealand. She did not take any drugs or traditional medicines during her entire trip. Her symptoms started two days after arrival in Singapore. She denied any rashes or respiratory symptoms. On examination, she was lethargic looking but orientated. Vital signs were temperature 42.2°C, heart rate 164/min, respiratory rate 22/min and blood pressure 103/65 mmHg.

Her initial blood investigations showed the following: haemoglobin 10.1 g/dL (12.0–16,0), white cell count 3.63 × 10(9)/L (4.0–10) and platelet count 99 × 10(9)/L (140–440). Her renal function and liver function tests were normal.

This was her electrocardiogram when she was experiencing a bout of palpitations at the time it was performed.

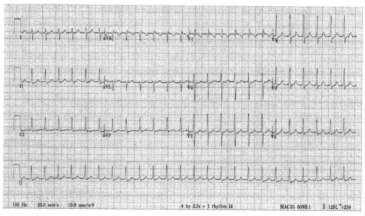

Image courtesy of Dr Chin Chee Yang.

1A. **Identify the cardiac rhythm.** (1 mark)

....

1B. **Name two drugs that can be administered to correct the rhythm.** (2 marks)

a. ....

b. ....

2. **Fill in the box below with your MOST likely differential diagnoses and an appropriate diagnostic investigation in this patient.** The first row has been completed for illustration.

	Differential Diagnosis ($1 \times 4 = 4$ marks)	Diagnostic Investigation ($1 \times 4 = 4$ marks)
A	Malaria	Malarial blood film
B		
C		
D		
E		

This was her blood film.

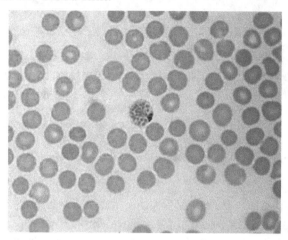

3.   What is the diagnosis?   (2 marks)

....

**4A. Which of the following is the MOST appropriate treat-
       ment?**   (2 marks)

    a. Artesunate monotherapy
    b. Artesunate + mefloquine
    c. Chloroquine monotherapy
    d. Chloroquine + doxycycline
    e. Hydroxychloroquine + clindamycin   (   )

4B. What additional treatment is necessary? Explain.
                                                    (2 marks)

....

....

A few months after recovery, the patient expressed interest to participate in a mission trip to Papua New Guinea.

5. **Suggest three MOST appropriate vaccinations or prophylaxis for this lady prior to her travel.** (3 marks)

a. ....

b. ....

c. ....

Question 2.3

A 40-year-old construction worker presented with a recurrent itchy rash on his upper limbs that has persisted for six months. Two weeks before seeing a doctor, he had applied some traditional Chinese medication to the rash, but it aggravated the rash instead.

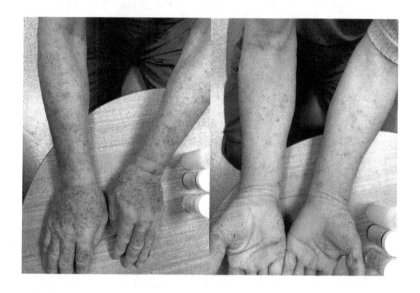

1. **Describe the morphology of the rash.**   (2 marks)

    ....

2. **What is the MOST likely diagnosis?**   (1 mark)

    ....

3. **Suggest two MOST likely aetiologies of the rash.**

(2 marks)

a. ....

b. ....

4. **Which of the following is the MOST appropriate investigation?** (2 marks)

   a. Patch testing
   b. Skin biopsy with direct immunofluorescence
   c. Skin biopsy with fungal culture
   d. Skin prick testing
   e. Skin scraping for microsopy ( )

5. **Which of the following management outcomes will MOST likely occur?** (1 mark)

   a. His condition is cured with a prolonged course of topical superpotent corticosteroid
   b. His condition is cured with a prolonged combination course of antibacterial and antifungal therapies
   c. His condition resolves with topical superpotent corticosteroid but recurs when he returns to work
   d. His condition resolves with a combination of antibacterial and antifungal therapies but recurs when he returns to work
   e. His condition is not responsive to topical superpotent corticosteroid, antibacterial or antifungal therapy ( )

About 20 years later, he is referred to the respiratory clinic after a chest X-ray to evaluate his shortness of breath. His chest radiograph is shown below:

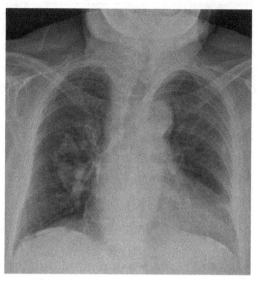

6A.   Identify two radiological abnormalities that are present in the X-ray.   (2 marks)

a. ....

b. ....

6B.   Suggest two radiological abnormalities, which may otherwise appear.   (2 marks)

a. ....

b. ....

7. **What three pertinent questions should you ask during history-taking?** (3 marks)

    a. ....

    b. ....

    c ....

8. **What is the MOST likely diagnosis? Justify.** (3 marks)

    ....

    ....

    ....

9. **Which of the following are the MOST useful diagnostic investigations? Choose TWO.** (2 marks)

    a. Bronchoscopy
    b. High-resolution CT thorax
    c. Pulmonary diffusion capacity
    d. Spirometry
    e. Sputum cytology
    f. Ventilation-perfusion scan   (   ) & (   )

Question 2.4

A 75-year-old man with a history of diabetes mellitus and hypertension presented with fever, chills and rigours for two days, associated with non-bilious vomiting. He was treated for a urinary tract infection about two weeks previously. Clinically, he was febrile with stable vital signs. His right kidney was ballotable and tender.

1A. Propose two differential diagnoses. (2 marks)

a. ....

b. ....

1B. Suggest another differential diagnosis had this patient NOT have fever, chills and rigours. (2 marks)

....

2. List six important aspects of history that you would like to ask that would impact evaluation and management.
(3 marks)

a. ....

b. ....

c. ....

d. ....

e. ....

f. ....

The following laboratory investigations were performed. Selected renal panel results from old records were also retrieved for trending.

	5 Jul 2018	16 Aug 2019	1 Oct 2019 (Admission)
Urea (2.7–6.9 mmol/L)	11.7	10.7	14.5
Sodium (136–146 mmol/L)	138	140	134
Potassium (3.5–5.1mmol/L)	4.8	5.1	4.1
Chloride (98–107 mmol/L)	102	104	99
Bicarbonate (19–29 mmol/L)	26.7	25	16.7
Creatinine (62–106 µmol/L)	186	173	227
CKD-EPI eGFR (mL/min)	30	33	23
Random Glucose (mmol/L)			11.0
Lipids (mmol/L)	Total cholesterol 2.24 HDL 0.83 Triglyceride 1.36 LDL 0.79		

3. Identify two key biochemical syndromes.   (2 marks)

a. ....

b. ....

A renal ultrasound was performed. The right kidney measured 19.0 cm, and the left, 16.9 cm. No hydronephrosis was reported.

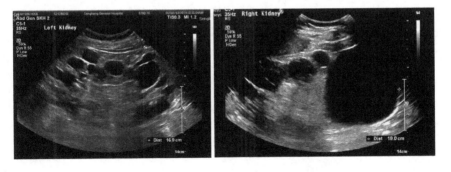

4.   Identify the radiological abnormalities.   (2 marks)

....

5.   Outline three principles of primary medical management of the patient.   (3 marks)

a. ....

b. ....

c. ....

6.   How would you educate the patient and his family?
          (4 marks)

....

....

....

....

In the middle of 2020, he presented to the emergency department with a headache. His blood pressure reading was 210/140 mmHg. Papilloedema was present on both fundi.

7.   Suggest two possible explanations for this development.
          (2 marks)

a. ....

b. ....

Question 2.5

A 50-year-old male was admitted to the hospital for left leg cellulitis. He had been diagnosed with hypertension and type 2 diabetes mellitus five years ago and is taking amlodipine 5 mg OM, enalapril 5 mg OM and metformin 500 mg BD. His height is 170 cm, and his weight is 80 kg. Except for the left leg inflammatory changes, his physical examination was unremarkable. The nurse requested that the patient be shifted to an individual room as his snoring (described as "like thunder") was disturbing his neighbours.

Below are his blood pressure readings (mmHg) since admission:

Day 1				Day 2				
8 am	12 pm	4 pm	8 pm	2 am	8 am	12 pm	4 pm	8 pm
160/98	143/90	155/78	150/88	140/88	165/78	145/99	151/98	143/83

Initial laboratory test results:

Urea, serum	3.2 mmol/L	(2.7–6.9)
Potassium, serum	2.8 mmol/L	(3.5–5.1)
Chloride, serum	101 mmol/L	(98–107)
Bicarbonate, serum	31 mmol/L	(19.0–29.0)
Glucose, serum	5.9 mmol/L	(3.9–11.0)
Creatinine, serum	59 μmol/L	(45–84)
Potassium, 24-hour urine	40 mol/day	

His electrocardiogram (ECG) and chest X-ray showed left ventricular hypertrophy.

1A. Which of the following are two MOST likely considerations in regard to the blood pressure readings?   (2 marks)

    a. Bartter syndrome
    b. Cushing syndrome
    c. Excessive Laxative intake
    d. Liddle syndrome
    e. Poor oral intake
    f. Primary aldosteronism
    g. Renal artery stenosis
    h. Renal tubular acidosis   (   ) & (   )

1B. Suggest a screening test and show how it distinguishes between these two.   (2 marks)

....

....

....

2A. Identify another possible cause for his secondary hypertension.   (2 marks)

....

2B. Suggest an appropriate investigation for this cause.   (1 mark)

....

The patient, on the morning of his third day of hospitalisation, was found to have profound right-sided weakness. He was able to follow instructions on eye movements (during which right homonymous hemianopia was detected). When asked whether he was experiencing pain or a loss of sensation, he replied with irrelevant words.

3A. **What is the MOST likely diagnosis?** (2 marks)

    a. Lacunar syndrome
    b. Partial anterior circulation syndrome
    c. Posterior circulation syndrome
    d. Total anterior circulation syndrome
    e. Weber syndrome   (   )

3B. **Identify the artery/arteries that is/are MOST likely to be affected.** (2 marks)

....

An urgent CT brain scan showed neither bleeding nor intraparen-chymal abnormality.

4. **Which of the following is the MOST appropriate manage-ment at this stage?** (2 marks)

    a. Oral antiplatelet therapy
    b. Intravenous thrombolysis with recombinant tissue plasmi-nogen activator
    c. Intravenous thrombolysis with streptokinase
    d. Initiation of oral anticoagulation
    e. Initiation of subcutaneous anticoagulation   (   )

5. **Suggest three useful investigations at this stage.**
                                    (3 marks)

    a. ....

    b. ....

    c. ....

6.   At what threshold should the blood pressure be treated?

(2 marks)

....

On day two after his stroke, the nurse called for an urgent review as the patient's blood pressure increased significantly.

Day 1 of Stroke				Day 2 of Stroke				
8 am	12 pm	4 pm	8 pm	2 am	8 am	12 pm	12.30 pm	1 pm
180/100	195/113	178/99	183/105	176/90	186/103	222/105	240/110	230/130

On review the patient appeared restless and uncomfortable. Physical examination revealed a palpable mass in his suprapubic region, which appeared to be tender on deep palpation.

7.   Outline your management to lower the patient's blood pressure.

(2 marks)

....

....

Assessment Paper
3

Question 3.1

A 78-year-old man presented at a general medicine clinic with a 2-week history of vertiginous giddiness and unsteady gait. Before this, he had a bout of upper respiratory tract infection with fever and decreased oral intake. His medical history comprised of ischaemic heart disease, diabetes mellitus, hypertension and benign prostatic hypertrophy. He is currently taking the following medications: aspirin 100 mg OM, metformin 500 mg TDS, glipizide 5 mg OM, atenolol 50 mg OM, enalapril 10 mg OM, tamsulosin 400 mcg ON. He is independent in his instrumental activities of daily living and continues to work at his long-term job as a petrol pump attendant.

Clinical examination showed mild cog-wheeling rigidity in his right upper limb. He was unsteady on his feet. His lying blood pressure was 105/72 mmHg, and his standing blood pressure was 82/55 mmHg (symptomatic).

1. **Suggest three MOST likely explanations for the blood pressure abnormality.** (3 marks)

   a. ....

   b. ....

   c. ....

2. **Apart from postural blood pressure, name three specific clinical assessments that should be performed in the clinic.** (3 marks)

a. ....

b. ....

c. ....

A decision was made to admit the patient from the clinic for further evaluation and management as he was likely to fall due to his giddiness and unsteady gait. Investigations were as follow:

Urea	12.4 mmol/L	(2.7–6.9)
Sodium	129 mmol/L	(136–146)
Potassium	4.8 mmol/L	(3.6–5.0)
Creatinine	144 µmol/L	(54–101)
Glucose	3.4 mmol/L	(3.9–6.0)
HbA1c	5.2%	

His electrocardiogram and chest X-ray were unremarkable.
A CT brain scan showed generalised cerebral atrophy.

3. **What are your three management priorities?** (3 marks)

a. ....

b. ....

c. ....

4. **Suggest a relevant blood investigation that you would order to be taken just before the patient's breakfast the next day.** (1 mark)

....

The patient was stabilised with the appropriate medical treatment, and his giddiness improved. He was able to ambulate more steadily though his gait was shuffling with reduced arm swing. He was keen to return to work.

5. **Name three pharmacological classes of drugs that could be considered for him.** (3 marks)

a. ....

b. ....

c. ....

The patient was started on a common fixed-dose combination drug for his gait-related issues. Shortly after starting treatment, he complained of giddiness. Again, a postural drop in blood pressure was documented.

6A. **Suggest two pharmacological strategies to manage this problem.** (2 marks)

a. ....

b. ....

6B. **Suggest two non-pharmacological strategies to manage this problem.** (2 marks)

a. ....

b. ....

During an outpatient visit, the patient also complained of an itchy rash on his face. He had been using a topical corticosteroid cream, which he took from a friend but with no improvement.

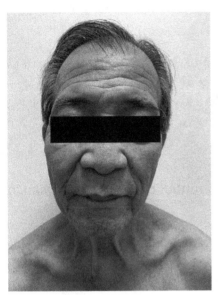 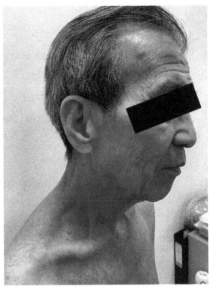

7. What is the MOST likely diagnosis? (2 marks)

    a. Allergic contact dermatitis

    b. Photoallergic drug reaction

    c. Phototoxic drug reaction

    d. Seborrhoeic dermatitis

    e. Tinea faciei. ( )

8. What complication has he developed due to applying the topical corticosteroid cream? (1 mark)

....

Question 3.2

A 50-year-old lady, who is an ex-smoker with no previous medical history, presented with pain of three days' duration over her foot. There was no history of trauma. Clinical examination showed a large red and tender swelling of the metatarsophalangeal joint of her left big toe.

1. **Give three MOST likely differential diagnoses.** (3 marks)

    a. ....

    b. ....

    c. ....

2. **Suggest two MOST appropriate diagnostic investigations.**
    (2 marks)

    a. ....

    b. ....

As part of the workup, these are her full blood count results:

Haemoglobin	19.6 g/dL	(14.0–18.0)
Mean Cell Volume	73.5 fL	(78.0–98.0)
Mean Cell Haemoglobin	21.1 pg	(27.0–32.0)

WBC Count $10.4 \times 10(9)/L$ (4–10)
Neutrophils $8.01 \times 10(9)/L$ (2.0–7.5)
Lymphocytes $1.28 \times 10(9)/L$ (1.0–3.0)
Monocytes $0.52 \times 10(9)/L$ (0.2–0.8)
Eosinophils $0.34 \times 10(9)/L$ (0.04–0.44)
Basophils $0.15 \times 10(9)/L$ (0–0.1)
Platelet Count $755 \times 10(9)/L$ (140–440)

3. **What is the MOST likely haematological diagnosis?**

(2 marks)

....

4. **Fill in the box below for differential diagnoses of the elevated haemoglobin. Row A has been completed for illustration purposes.**   (0.5 x 4 = 2 marks)

	Aetiological Category	Specific Clinical Example
A	Exogenous erythropoietin (EPO)	Surreptitious self-injections to enhance athletic performance
B		
C		

The patient also mentioned that she had been having intermittent headaches for the past two months and occasionally had red painful fingers, with no particular pattern to the episodes. Each episode lasted for one to two hours. This is a photograph taken when the redness occurred:

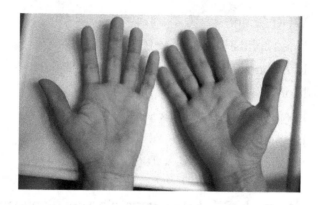

5A. Identify the clinical phenomenon.   (1 mark)

....

5B. Explain its pathogenesis in the clinical context of this patient.   (2 marks)

....

....

Numerous diagnostic investigations were performed.

6.   What is the key histological feature in a bone marrow biopsy?   (1 mark)

....

7.   Give two suitable pharmacological therapies for this patient.   (2 marks)

a. ....

b. ....

After having her joint problem resolved, the patient defaulted on her follow-up. Two years later, she re-presented with joint pains in her hands.

This is a photograph of a different patient showing similar findings as hers.

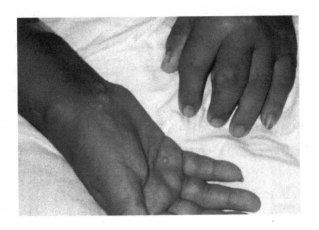

8. **Describe the abnormalities observed.**   (2 marks)

    ....

    ....

The clinician decided to start her on allopurinol when the acute pain subsided.

9. **Give three precautions that should be taken when this decision is made.**   (3 marks)

    a. ....

    b. ....

    c. ....

Question 3.3

A 35-year-old male technician attended a basic health screening. His medical history was significant for recently diagnosed hypertension (blood pressure 150/90 mmHg on two occasions) and bilateral carpal tunnel syndrome a year ago, managed conservatively by a private orthopaedic surgeon. He does not smoke cigarettes or consume alcohol beverages. He has no family history of hypertension, hyperlipidaemia or diabetes mellitus.

Clinical examination revealed an overweight man of weight 86 kg and height 178 cm. His blood pressure reading was 160/95 mmHg, and pulse rate, 70/min. Chest auscultation revealed normal dual heart sounds and no murmur. Respiratory and abdominal examinations were unremarkable.

1.   In the context of the above history, what further aspects of the cardiovascular system would you make an effort to examine? (2 marks)

....

....

The following observations were also noted.

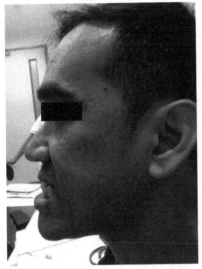 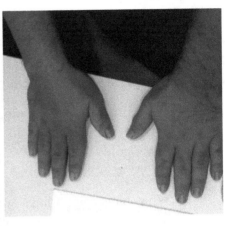

2.   Identify three physical features that may be of clinical significance.   (3 marks)

a. ....

b. ....

c. ....

These are his serial facial photographs.

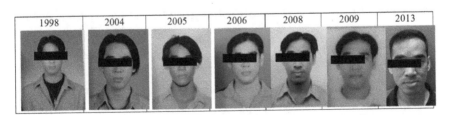

3.   **Identify one progressive physical sign change in the serial photographs that you have not described in Question 2.**   (1 mark)

    ....

4.   **To complete your physical examination:**

    A. What important **neurological** examination would you perform to elucidate an underlying pathophysiological abnormality?   (1 mark)

    ....

    B. What physical findings would you look for in the **neck**, which relate to a hormonal connection?   (2 marks)

    ....

In the diagnostic workup of this patient, a young medical student suggested checking the random growth hormone level.

5.   **What is your reply to him?**   (1 mark)

    ....

    ....

Instead, an oral glucose tolerance test with serial measurements of the growth hormone and insulin-like growth factor-1 (IGF-1) was performed.

	Normal ranges/ units	0 min	30 min	60 min	90 min	120 min	150 min
GH	0.16–13 mIU/L	14.8	12.8	15.2	11.0	13.4	16.2
Glucose	3.1–7.8 mmol/L	5.5	8.5	8.3	6.8	5.4	4.6
IGF-1	109–284 ng/ml	536	—	—	—	—	—

6. What is your interpretation of these results? (3 marks)

....

....

....

You also noted from the health screen results that the serum calcium levels were elevated at 2.80 mmol/L (2.10–2.60).

7. What is the next MOST appropriate investigation?

(1 mark)

....

8. What is the MOST appropriate advice concerning genetic testing? (2 marks)

a. It is not indicated.
b. It should be offered to detect a mutation in familial hypocalciuric hypercalcaemia
c. It should be offered to detect a mutation in the multiple endocrine neoplasia type 1 gene (MEN 1 gene)
d. It should be offered to detect a mutation in the multiple endocrine neoplasia type 2 gene (RET protooncogene)
e. It should be offered to detect a mutation in the Von Hippel–Lindau syndrome. (   )

The MRI of his brain showed a pituitary adenoma.

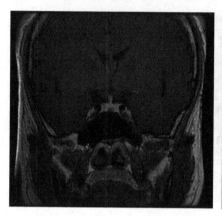 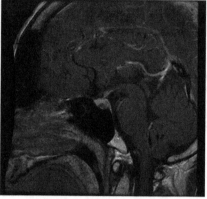

9.   Mark the abnormality on each image.   (0.5 x 2 marks)

10.   If the patient declined trans-sphenpoidal surgery, propose two treatment options.   (2 marks)

a. ....

b. ....

During a follow-up visit, the patient complained of frequent constipation.

11.   What is the MOST appropriate investigation?   (1 mark)

....

Question 3.4

A 70-year-old man, recently diagnosed with lung cancer with metastases to his bones, liver and lymph nodes, was on best supportive care. He was admitted with a 2-day history of confusion and agitation. His disorientation was observed to fluctuate throughout the day. He would become agitated at times and drowsy at other times. On examination, he was awake and able to talk, but not able to answer questions. His vital signs showed a blood pressure of 100/64 mmHg, pulse rate of 98/min and oxygen saturation 93% on room air.

You want to check for uraemia, hyponatraemia and hypercalcaemia, which might account for this sudden change in mentation.

1. **Suggest three *other* MOST likely explanations for the acute confusion apart from these considerations.**
    (3 marks)

    a. ....

    b. ....

    c. ....

You found a possible cause for his acute confusional state and started treatment for it. However, the patient remained agitated and was observed by the nurses as constantly trying to climb out of his bed.

2.   Suggest one:

A. Pharmacological measure   (1 mark)

....

B. Non-pharmacological measure   (1 mark)

....

The patient continued to deteriorate despite optimal medical treatment, likely due to the progression of an underlying disease. He has become lethargic and barely responsive. You diagnose that the patient is dying.

3.   Give three management principles at this stage.

                                                       (3 marks)

a. ....

b. ....

c. ....

The patient is actively dying; he is barely responsive and unable to express his wishes. As the primary medical team, you have judged that in the event of cardiorespiratory collapse, cardiopulmonary resuscitation (CPR) would be futile. The next-of-kin understands the poor prognosis but insists nonetheless that "everything should be done to try to save him" and demands that CPR be performed.

4.   What is the correct course of action and MOST appropriate ethical justification?   (2 marks)

a. CPR should be done because the patient is not able to decline it.

b. CPR should be done because the patient has lost capacity, so the next-of-kin makes the final decision, after having considered recommendations from the medical team.

    c. CPR should be done to avoid a complaint from the family.

    d. CPR should not be done because the primary medical team makes the final decision, after having considered the patient's and family's wishes.

    e. Full CPR should not be done, but a "gentle form" of CPR can be performed so that the next-of-kin's wishes can be accommodated.   ( )

The family subsequently showed the medical team an advance care planning (ACP) document that was completed a year ago by the patient. This document stated that "(the patient) wanted to live for as long as possible, and to continue trying all medical treatments, even if (my) chance of recovery is low".

5. **With this ACP document, what is the correct course of action and MOST appropriate ethical justification?**

                                        (2 marks)

    a. CPR should be done because this is consistent with the patient's previously expressed wishes.

    b. CPR should be done because the patient has lost capacity, so the next-of-kin makes the final decision, after having considered recommendations from the medical team.

    c. CPR should be done because the ACP document is legally binding.

    d. CPR should not be done because the primary medical team makes the final decision, after having considered the patient's and family's wishes.

    e. Full CPR should not be done, but a "gentle form" of CPR can be performed so that the next-of-kin's wishes can be accommodated.   ( )

After further discussion, the family is now agreeable with comfort measures and not for CPR. However, they request for artificial hydration and nutrition so that the patient will not "starve to death".

6.   **Name two medical, social and/or ethical considerations when navigating this issue of artificial hydration and nutrition at the patient's end of life.**   (2 marks)

a. ....

b. ....

It is decided that a trial of intravenous fluid will be given to the patient. The next day, the patient deteriorates further, with increasing respiratory tract secretions that result in a "rattling" sound when the patient breathes.

7.   **Suggest one:**

A. Pharmacological measure to cope with the secretions
(1 mark)

....

B. Non-pharmacological measure to cope with the secretions
(1 mark)

....

The next day, the patient's respiratory tract secretions are lessened; however, he starts to become more restless — grimacing and groaning intermittently. He remains very lethargic; he opens his eyes to the sound of voices but has no eye contact or meaningful communication. On examination, the patient does not appear to have any symptoms and signs to suggest a specific case of restlessness. His blood pressure is 90/54 mmHg, pulse rate 110/min and oxygen saturation 95% on 4L/min oxygen via nasal prongs.

8. **What is the next MOST appropriate management?**

   (2 marks)

   a. Administer 500 ml of intravenous fluid to increase his blood pressure
   b. Administer a stat dose of subcutaneous haloperidol to treat his restlessness
   c. Arrange for a CT brain scan to rule out an intracranial event
   d. Blood investigations including full blood count and renal function
   e. Start morphine infusion as the patient is dying   (   )

The patient is now comfortable but continues to deteriorate generally.

9. **Give two clinical signs to suggest that the patient is actively dying.** (2 marks)

   a. ....

   b. ....

Question 3.5

A 50-year-old Chinese fish farmer presented at the emergency department with severe pain and swelling of his right leg, associated with a fever of one day's duration. He has a background history of diabetes (a check from the system showed his latest HbA1c to be 13%). He smokes twenty sticks of cigarettes and consumes five to eight bottles of beer daily. He recalled developing a mild rash when he was prescribed penicillin in the past. His vital signs were: temperature 38.7°C, blood pressure 120/80 mmHg, pulse rate 90/min and respiratory rate 16/min. His right foot and calf were oedematous, erythematous, warm and tender.

An hour later, upon reaching the general ward, he became very lethargic. His vital signs were: temperature 38.5°C, blood pressure 80/40 mmHg, pulse rate 110/min and respiratory rate 22/min. The extent of the swelling had extended well beyond a line drawn over the right calf at the emergency department. Close observation revealed a small fish hook embedded in the webspace between the first and second toes of his right foot. The rest of the physical examination was unremarkable.

1. **Propose two pathophysiological explanations for the tachypnea.** (2 marks)

    a. ....

    b. ....

2. **List five *immediate* management principles.**   (5 marks)

   a. ....

   b. ....

   c. ....

   d. ....

   e. ....

3. **Outline how would you improve the blood pressure:**

   A. In the general ward now.   (2 marks)

   ....

   ....

   B. If the above is unsuccessful.   (2 marks)

   ....

   ....

4. **List two additional specific aspects that you would look for in the patient's health records that may impact his management.**   (2 marks)

   a. ....

   b. ....

5. **Propose a specific plan on:**

   A. Pharmacological treatment for his condition.   (2 marks)

   ....

   ....

B. Non-pharmacological treatment for his condition.

(2 marks)

....

....

Upon the patient's recovery, you seek to evaluate his history of possible penicillin allergy.

6. List three specific questions that are helpful: (3 marks)

a. ....

b. ....

c. ....

Assessment Paper

4

Question 4.1

A 45-year-old man was admitted after he accidentally rolled off the sofa. He was extremely overweight with very limited movements — he only moved to go to the toilet, while the rest of his time was spent lying on the sofa or eating on his bed.

He has a history of diabetes (his last HbA1c was 8% five years ago) and was never compliant with medication. He was also a Hepatitis B carrier. He was a non-smoker and did not consume alcohol. He lived alone, and his siblings brought food to him three times daily.

1. **Suggest two reasons why this patient may be prone to falls.** (2 marks)

   a. ....

   b. ....

On examination, his body weight was 180 kg with a body mass index of 59 kg/m^2. His vital signs were: temperature 36.0°C, blood pressure 110/80 mmHg, heart rate 90/min and oxygen saturation 99% on room air. His heart sounds were dual, and breath sounds were vesicular. A neurological examination was difficult; his power was full on all four limbs.

2. **Name two cutaneous signs on an *abdominal examination* that you would look for in each of these groups:**

A. That suggest an underlying organic cause for the obesity.

(2 marks)

a. ....

b. ....

B. That are a complication of the obesity. (2 marks)

a. ....

b. ....

All the signs in Question 2A were absent on closer examination. Preliminary relevant laboratory investigations were as follow:

Haemoglobin	11.7 g/dL	(14–18)
WBC Count	$4.0 \times 10(9)/L$	(4–10)
Platelet Count	$70 \times 10(9)/L$	(140–440)
Blood Urea	7.0 mmol/L	(4.7–6.9)
Sodium	130 mmol/L	(135–145)
Potassium	4.0 mmol/L	(3.5–4.5)
Serum Creatinine	80 µmol/L	(60–104)
Total Bilirubin	19 mmol/L	(7–32)
Aspartate Transaminase	13 U/L	(6–66)
Alkaline Phosphatase	109 U/L	(39–99)
Alanine Transaminase	27 U/L	(12–42)
HbA1c	5.6%	

3. **What would be the MOST likely unifying explanation for these laboratory abnormalities in this patient?** (2 marks)

    ....

    ....

4. **Propose an explanation for the "spontaneous" improvement in HbA1c.** (1 mark)

    ....

5. **Name three clinical signs on an *abdominal* examination that you would look for in this patient in the light of the findings and conclusions.** (3 marks)

    a. ....

    b. ....

    c. ....

A further abdominal examination did not reveal any of these abnormalities.

6. **Suggest four further investigations to guide diagnosis and treatment of the condition related to his Hepatitis B:**

    A. Laboratory   (2 marks)

    a. ....

    b. ....

    B. Imaging   (2 marks)

    a. ....

    b. ....

The patient was discharged against medical advice. He was read-mitted six years later when he presented with acute confusion of one week's duration. He appeared markedly pale with a severely distended and tender abdomen. He also demonstrated asterixis.

7. **Suggest two MOST plausible explanations for the confusion.** (2 × 2 = 4 marks)

    a. ....

    ....

    b. ....

    ....

Question 4.2

A 48-year-old obese housewife complained of an itchy rash on her chest and back for a few months. She had been treated by her general practitioner (GP) with a topical clotrimazole 1% cream with no effect. She has a background of chronic hypertension on follow-ups with her GP.

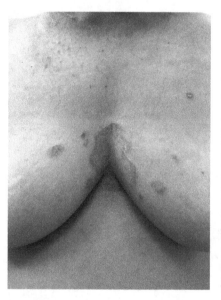 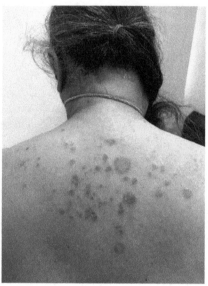

1.   **Describe the rash.**   (2 marks)

....

2.   **Where on her body would you specifically like to look for a similar rash? Select the area(s) with the highest yield.**
     (2 marks)

   a.   Anogenitalia
   b.   Axillae and groins
   c.   Buccal mucosa
   d.   Elbows and knees
   e.   Palms and soles   (   )

3.   **Pertaining to the evolution of this rash, which aspect of her history would you be interested to find out?** (2 marks)

   a.   Alcohol consumption
   b.   Blood pressure control
   c.   Menstrual status
   d.   Sexual activity
   e.   Weight changes   (   )

Examination of her hands showed the following.

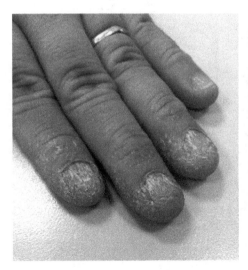
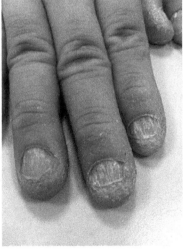

4.   Which of the following conditions is the MOST likely diagnosis?   (2 marks)

    a. Atopic eczema
    b. Irritant contact dermatitis
    c. Onychomycosis
    d. Psoriasis
    e. Viral warts   (   )

5.   Suggest two specific abnormalities that you may observe on her toenails.   (2 marks)

    a. ....

    b. ....

On two previous occasions, her left second toe became painfully swollen. This is a photograph of the feet of a different patient depicting similar findings.

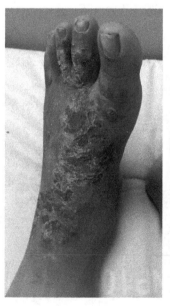 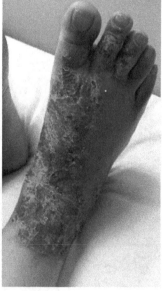

6A. **What is the MOST likely explanation?** (1 mark)

....

6B. **Which of the following would be the MOST appropriate treatment in this situation?** (2 marks)

   a. Colchicine
   b. Diclofenac
   c. Physiotherapy
   d. Prednisolone
   e. Warm compresses   ( )

6C. **In which of the following conditions can this phenomenon also be seen?** (1 mark)

   a. Ankylosing spondylitis
   b. Osteomyelitis
   c. Rheumatoid arthritis
   d. Secondary syphilis
   e. Thalassaemia major   ( )

7. **To complete a targeted and holistic physical examination, which of the following areas would be the LEAST important?** (2 marks)

   a. Body mass index
   b. Conjunctivae
   c. Mood
   d. Sacroiliac joint
   e. Thyroid gland   ( )

After discussing the options and performing the necessary baseline tests, the patient was commenced on oral ciclosporin. Three weeks later, she returned with a significant flaring of her condition. Her entire body was red and flaky, and she was shivering in a wheelchair.

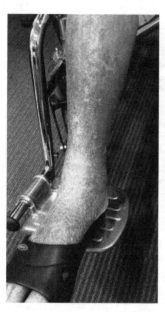 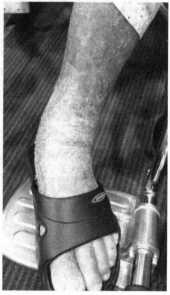

8A. Propose two possible explanations for this development.
(2 marks)

a. ....

b. ....

8B. Outline two management principles.   (2 marks)

a. ....

b. ....

Question 4.3

A 60-year-old man presented with bilateral lower limb swelling for the past two weeks associated with reduced effort tolerance and chest tightness for a day. He has a history of type 2 diabetes mellitus for four years with non-proliferative diabetic retinopathy in both eyes, hypertension, hyperlipidemia and a past history of left Bell's palsy.

1. **For each of the suspected aetiologies grouped as follows, state two symptoms that you would ask for.**

   A. Cardiac   (2 marks)

   a. ....

   b. ....

   B. Renal   (2 marks)

   a. ....

   b. ....

On clinical examination, his vital signs were: temperature 35.6°C, blood pressure 183/99 mmHg, regular heart rate 89/min, respiratory rate 19/min and oxygen saturation 98% on room air. He had bilateral lower limb pitting edema to the knees. The jugular venous pressure was not raised. Chest auscultation revealed no heart murmurs and very minimal basal crepitations.

2.   In pursuit of the clinical diagnosis, what clinical signs would you specifically look for in this patient? (2 marks)

....

....

These were his initial laboratory investigations:

Haemoglobin	10.5 g/dL	(14–18)
WBC Count	6.12 × 10(9)/L	(4–10)
Platelet Count	244 × 10(9)/L	(140–440)
MCV	81.2 fL	(78.0–98.0)
MCH	29.0 pg	(27.0–32.0)
RBC Distribution Width	12.6%	(10.9–15.7)
Blood Urea	7.1 mmol/L	(2.7–6.9)
Sodium	139 mmol/L	(136–146)
Potassium	4.0 mmol/L	(3.5–5.1)
Bicarbonate	25.0 mmol/L	(19.0–29.0)
Chloride	100 mmol/L	(98–107)
Serum Creatinine*	165 µmol/L	(62–106)
CKD-EPI, eGFR	39 mL/min/1.73 m^2	
Creatinine Kinase-MB	3.0 µg/L	(1.0–5.0)
Troponin T	42 ng/L	(≤29)

*Serum creatinine levels checked 6, 8 and 14 months ago were 133 µmol/L, 116 µmol/L and 112µmol/L, respectively.

Chest x-ray report: Heart size is at the upper limits of normal. No focal consolidation, pleural effusion or pneumothorax.

This is his electrocardiogram (ECG):

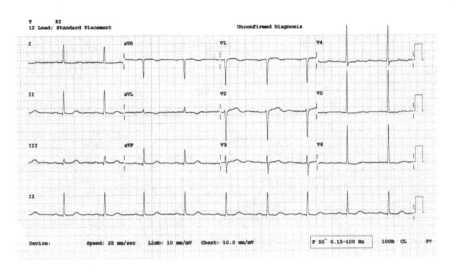

3. **In the light of a suspected cardiac aetiology comment on the ECG findings.** (2 marks)

....

....

4. **Comment on the troponin T result in the context of this patient.** (1 mark)

....

....

Additional investigations showed:

Urine	RBC	5/uL	(0–4)
	WBC	28/uL	(0–6)
	Epithelial Cell	0/uL	(0–4)
	Casts	Not seen	
	Crystals	Not seen	
	Microorganism	Not seen	
	Creatinine	11,460 μmol/L	
	Total Protein	>6.00 g/L	

Urine Protein: Creatinine ratio cannot be reliably calculated because urine protein is above the detection limit of the assay.

Serum Albumin	31 g/L	(35–50)
Total Cholesterol	3.03 mmol/L	(<5.2)
LDL Cholesterol	1.12	(<2.6)
HBs Ag	Positive	
Anti-HBs	Negative	

5.   Specific a urine test to order.   (1 mark)

....

6.   Summarise the clinical syndrome(s) in this patient's current presentation.   (2 marks)

....

....

7. **Give two MOST likely differential diagnoses for the aetiology in this patient.** (2 marks)

    a. ....

    b. ....

An ultrasound of his abdomen showed a smooth liver outline and parenchymal echotexture. Both kidneys had a normal echo pattern. The right kidney measured 11.70 cm and the left 10.40 cm in bipolar length. He was planned for an ultrasound-guided kidney biopsy.

8. **Give two prerequisities that should be fulfilled before scheduling the patient for a kidney biopsy.** (2 marks)

    a. ....

    b. ....

The histology of the kidney biopsy was reported as diabetic nephropathy and malignant nephrosclerosis.

9. **Outline four management principles that you would adopt for this patient.** (0.5 × 4 = 2 marks)

    a. ....

    b. ....

    c. ....

    d. ....

Upon discharge from the hospital, the patient's medications included irbesartan, bisoprolol, frusemide, terazosin, atorvastatin and linagliptin. His renal panel on review in six months showed the following:

Blood Urea	17.8 mmol/L	(2.7–6.9)
Sodium	134 mmol/L	(136–146)
Potassium	5.2 mmol/L	(3.5–5.1)
Bicarbonate	18.4 mmol/L	(19.0–29.0)
Chloride	105 mmol/L	(98–107)
Serum Creatinine	266 µmol/L	(62–106)
CKD-EPI, eGFR	22 mL/min/1.73m^2	

10. Suggest two explanations for the hyperkalaemia.

(2 marks)

a. ....

b. ....

Question 4.4

A 59-year-old male presented to the clinic with an unsteady gait over the past two years.

This is a photograph of part of his lower limbs.

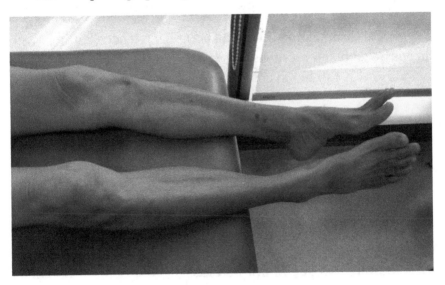

1. **Describe the important clinical findings.**   (2 marks)

    ....

    ....

2.   Based on your observations, what diagnosis should be considered? (1 mark)

....

3.   In the history-taking, what aspects pertaining to diet and lifestyle would be relevant in this context? Give two. (2 marks)

a. ....

b. ....

A physical examination revealed absent deep tendon reflexes with an equivocal plantar response as well as a loss of position sense.
    This is his full blood count done by his general practitioner:

Haemoglobin	10.9 g/dL	(12–16)
WBC Count	$2.96 \times 10(9)/L$	(4–10)
Platelet Count	$120 \times 10(9)/L$	(140–440)
MCV	113.4 fL	(78.0–98.0)
MCH	37.6 pg	(27.1–32.4)
RBC Distribution Width	14.9%	(12.2–14.8)

4A.   Identify two key abnormalities. (2 marks)

a. ....

b. ....

4B.   What is the MOST likely haematologic diagnosis? (2 marks)

....

Additional tests revealed the following:

Serum Cholesterol	3.54 mmol/L	(<5.2)
Serum Triglycerides	0.85 mmol/L	(1.7–2.2)
Serum Cholesterol, HDL	1.39 mmol/L	(1.0–1.5)
LDL (Calculated)	1.77 mmol/L	(2.6–3.3)
Serum Folate	22 mmol/L	(9–61)
Serum B12	100 pmol/L	(145–569)

5. **In the light of these findings, suggest an explanation for the high mean corpuscular haemoglobin (MCH).** (1 mark)

....

6. **Suggest two additional relevant laboratory investigations in this patient.** (2 marks)

a. ....

b. ....

7. **Postulate the reason(s) for the relatively low lipid levels compared to the general population?** (2 marks)

....

....

The patient declared he was a complete vegetarian.

8. **What is your unifying diagnosis?** (2 marks)

....

9. **In the diagram of the spinal cord shade the respective affected areas in this patient.** (2 marks)

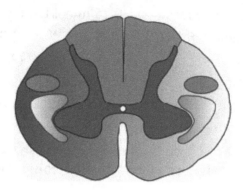

10. **Suggest two positive neurological signs that might be elicited in this patient.** (2 marks)

    a. ....

    b. ....

Question 4.5

A 65-year-old female was admitted for two episodes of transient loss of consciousness (TLoC) over the past one month. Her past medical history includes hypertension, hyperlipidaemia, poorly-controlled type 2 diabetes mellitus (HbA1c 9% one month ago), a "mild" lacunar stroke two months ago, and previous radiotherapy for a "cancer" ten years ago. Her current medications are amlodipine 10 mg OM, telmisartan 80 mg OM, atenolol 50 mg OM, prazosin 2 mg BD, atorvastatin 40 mg ON, metformin 850 mg BD, linagliptin 5 mg OM, and aspirin 100 mg OM.

On examination, her cardiovascular, respiratory and abdominal systems were unremarkable. A neurological examination revealed mild weakness in the right upper and lower limbs, and reduced sensation affecting both her hands and feet. She could not articulate her words clearly, and the speech therapist had assessed her to have moderate oropharyngeal dysphagia.

1. **Give four MOST likely differential diagnoses for her TLoC.**

   (4 marks)

   a. ....

   b. ....

   c. ....

   d. ....

According to the son who witnessed both episodes of loss of consciousness, there was no limb jerking, tongue biting, urinary or bowel incontinence. She regained consciousness fairly quickly afterwards.

2. **Suggest two bedside investigations or manoeuvres that may elicit the cause of her TLoC?**   (2 marks)

     a. ....

     b. ....

Below are her blood pressure readings on the first day of admission:

	Day 1							
	8 am	8.02 am	8.03 am	12 pm	12.03 pm	8 pm	8.01 pm	8.03 pm
Lying BP (Heart Rate)	140/99 (65)			130/80 (56)		135/90 (62)		
Sitting BP (Heart Rate)		125/95 (64)					122/83 (60)	
Standing BP (Heart Rate)			101/91 (68)		95/70 (60)			105/79 (65)

3A. **Interpret the blood pressure readings.**   (1 mark)

....

3B. **Propose two MOST likely causes for the interpretation.**   (2 marks)

     a. ....

     b. ....

The next morning, a short Synacthen Test (SST) was performed as part of an evaluation of hyponatraemia. An intravenous injection of 250 mcg of Synacthen was given at 8.01 am. Below are the results:

Time	8 am	8.31 am	9.01 am
ACTH (ng/L) Normal Range: 10.0–60.0	5.5	N/A	N/A
Serum Cortisol (nmol/L)	140	250	300

4. What is your interpretation of the results? (3 marks)

....

....

As part of a workup for the peripheral neuropathy, her thyroid function was checked: serum free thyroxine (T4) was 9.1 pmol/L (12.7–20.3), and serum thyroid-stimulating hormone was 0.410 mIU/L (0.701–4.280). Her Vitamin B12 level was also low.

5A. What is your interpretation of the thyroid function result? (1 mark)

....

5B. Provide a unifying explanation for the conclusions drawn from the short Synacthen test and thyroid function test in this patient. (3 marks)

....

....

6.   Which of the following drugs may be a cause of the Vitamin B12 deficiency?   **(1 mark)**

    a. Aspirin
    b. Atenolol
    c. Atorvastatin
    d. Metformin
    e. Telmisartan   (   )

7.   Which of the following is the MOST important management priority for this patient at this stage?   **(1 mark)**

    a. Cerebral electrophysiological evaluation
    b. Optimisation of thyroid replacement
    c. Optimisation of glucocorticoid replacement
    d. Normalisation of blood pressure
    e. Speech and swallowing evaluation   (   )

During the multidisciplinary ward round, the consultant observed that the patient was very hard of hearing. An otoscopy performed at the bedside showed an intact tympanic membrane.

8.   Suggest two MOST likely explanations for the presbycusis.
                                                                 (2 marks)

    a. ....

    b. ....

Assessment Paper

5

Question 5.1

An ambulance was called after a 44-year-old businessman vomited a large pool of blood while singing at a karaoke club. On arrival, the paramedics found him in a confused and dazed state with a large pool of bloody vomitus on the floor. The only quick history the paramedics obtained from the hostesses was that he was their regular customer, and that he could drink and sing for hours. Recently, he started to forget the names of some of the hostesses he was fairly acquainted with.

On examination in the emergency department, his vital signs were: temperature 37.7°C, pulse rate 130/min, blood pressures 99/60 mmHg (lying down) and 80/50 mmHg (sitting up). His Glasgow Coma Scale (GCS) was 9/15 (E2, S3, M4), and he smelt of alcohol, cigarette smoke and vomit. There was clotted blood around his lips and mouth. Multiple spider telangiectasias were seen on his chest. Central Nervous System (CNS) examination was difficult due to his fluctuating conscious level and inability to cooperate. On fleeting moments of GCS 15/15, nystagmus was observed. His abdomen was distended. A rectal examination showed fresh and old blood on the glove; no masses or haemorrhoids were present.

These are his hands:

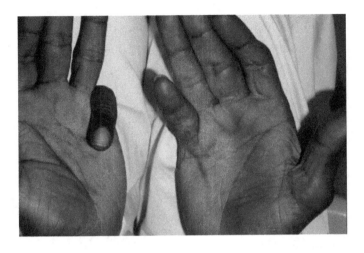

1. **Identify two abnormalities seen.** (2 marks)

a. ....

b. ....

2. **What other *useful* physical signs would you look for on the *hands*?** (2 marks)

....

....

3. **Suggest three plausible causes of his altered mental state.** (3 marks)

a. ....

b. ....

c. ....

These are his initial laboratory investigations:

Haemoglobin	9.0 g/dL	(14–18)
WBC Count	12.0 × 10(9)/L	(4–10)
Platelet Count	130 × 10(9)/L	(150–450)
MCV	97 fL	(76–96)
Prothrombin Time	15 sec	(9.9–11.4)
APTT	31 sec	(25.7–32.9)
Blood Urea	12 mmol/L	(4.7–6.9)
Sodium	131 mmol/L	(135–145)
Potassium	3.8 mmol/L	(3.5–5.3)
Serum Creatinine	99 μmol/L	(65–125)
Total Bilirubin	31 mmol/L	(5–30)
Albumin	32 mmol/L	(37–51)
Alkaline Phosphatase	104 U/L	(32–102)
Aspartate Transaminase	230 U/L	(10–45)
Alanine Transaminase	101 U/L	(10–55)
Gamma GT	324 U/L	(9–53)

A peripheral blood smear showed round macrocytes. Hypersegmented neutrophils were not seen.

4.   **Suggest two MOST likely causes for the macrocytosis.**
                                                                    (2 marks)

a. ....

b. ....

5. **Which of the following are life-saving management steps at this stage? Select four.** (4 marks)

a. Emergency gastroscopy
b. Endotracheal intubation
c. Fleet enema
d. Intravenous ceftriaxone
e. Intravenous mannitol
f. Intravenous terlipressin
g. Intravenous thiamine
h. Intravenous Vitamin K
i. Oral lactulose
j. Oxygen by non-rebreather mask
k. Transfusion of packed cells
l. Transfusion of
   platelets ( ) & ( ) & ( ) & ( )

6. **What further investigations could be performed to investigate his altered mental state?**

A Give two blood tests. (2 marks)
a. ....

b. ....

B Give two other tests. (2 marks)
a. ....

b. ....

He was subsequently diagnosed as having oesophageal variceal bleed due to alcoholic liver disease and dry beriberi.

7.   **Give three MOST useful recommendations to prevent a recurrence of his presenting symptoms.**   (3 marks)

   a. ....

   b. ....

   c. ....

Question 5.2

A 41-year-old lady presented with eye pain and blurred vision for two days. The pain was worse in her left eye and worse when looking at bright light. She described seeing floaters and flickering lights. On the first day, she also experienced headache, neck ache, giddiness and nausea. Her medical history was notable for diabetes mellitus (HbA1c 8.3% one year ago), hyperlipidaemia and hypothyroidism on replacement therapy. She recently saw a gynaecologist for menorrhagia with mild iron-deficiency anaemia. She was married with two children, aged 19 and 14.

On clinical examination, her vital signs were normal. Her conjunctivae were not inflamed, and her eye movements were full. Her neck was supple, and no focal neurology was demonstrated.

1. **Give two MOST important differential diagnoses that should be considered.** (2 marks)

    a. ....

    b. ....

A fundoscopy showed bilateral grossly swollen optic discs.

**2.   Which of the following is the next MOST appropriate
        investigation?**   (2 marks)

    a. CT brain scan
    b. Fluorescein angiography
    c. HbA1c
    d. Intraocular pressure assessment
    e. Lumbar puncture   (   )

**3.   What important clinical monitoring should be performed
        regularly? List three.**   (3 marks)

    a. ....

    b. ....

    c. ....

During the ward round on the second day of admission, diplopia on
horizontal gaze on her left side was demonstrated.

4.   What is the clinical *significance* of this new finding?
                                                           (1 mark)

....

An MRI brain scan was performed. It showed a loss of flow signal
in the left transverse sinus, sigmoid sinus, and the left internal jugular vein, in keeping with extensive venous sinus thrombosis.

5. **Give four important aspects of history in relation to** *aetiology* **that you would take from the patient.** (4 marks)

    a. ....

    b. ....

    c. ....

    d. ....

6. **What investigations, in relation to aetiology, would you order?**

    A. Laboratory — antibody test(s)   (2 marks)

    ....

    ....

    B. Laboratory — genetic test(s)   (2 marks)

    ....

    C. Radiological   (2 marks)

    ....

    ....

Anticoagulation was initiated. The patient was concerned as she recently developed menorrhagia.

7. **What blood test would you order in relation to a possible cause of her menorrhagia?**   (2 marks)

    ....

Question 5.3

A 34-year-old driver presented to his general practitioner with symptoms of dyspnoea, irritability and a loss of weight of 5 kg over three weeks. He had a neck swelling that moved upwards with swallowing. He was a smoker of 10 pack-years and drank 1–2 cans of beer every day. His thyroid function test confirmed thyrotoxicosis.

This is a photograph of his eyes:

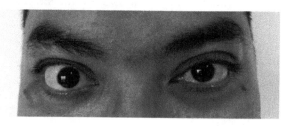

1A. Identify the abnormality. (1 mark)

....

1B. What observable complication of this abnormality is not seen here? (1 mark)

....

2. **What signs are you likely to elicit upon *palpation* of the neck swelling?** (2 marks)

   ....

   ....

3. **What signs are you likely to detect on examination of the hands?** (2 marks)

   ....

   ....

4. **What diagnostic investigation would you perform?** (1 mark)

   ....

The doctor considered starting the patient on carbimazole 30 mg once a day.

5. **Name two MOST useful tests that you would perform if suspecting a side-effect from this treatment.** (2 marks)

   a. ....

   b. ....

6. **What is the MOST important lifestyle advice that you would give to this patient?** (2 marks)

   ....

This patient was not compliant to his carbimazole and presented two years later with worsening dyspnoea, palpitations and another 4 kg of weight loss. His eyes looked the same as before. Cardiac auscultation revealed a scratchy sound on the left sternal border.

7.   Suggest one explanation for the auscultatory finding.
                                                                    (1 mark)

....

8.   What other abnormalities would you look out for in the cardiovascular examination? **(2 marks)**

....

....

He was found to be biochemically hyperthyroid. This is his electrocardiogram:

9A. Identify the electrocardiographic abnormalities. (1 mark)

....

9B. Which of the following is the MOST appropriate management for this disorder at this stage? (2 marks)

    a. Anticoagulation
    b. Beta-blocker
    c. Cardioversion
    d. Observation
    e. Systemic corticosteroid   (   )

After this episode, the patient was compliant with his treatment. On review at the clinic four weeks later, his symptoms have considerably improved, and his thyroid function has normalised. However, he has developed a painful rash on his legs as well as painful swollen ankles.

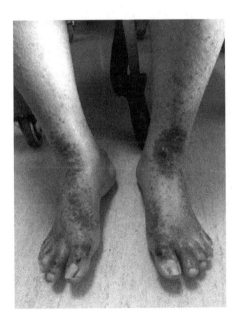

10. In the context of his thyroid condition, suggest an explanation for this eruption. (1 mark)

....

The doctor discusses the definitive treatments available for his thyroid condition.

11.   Which definitive treatment for his thyroid condition would you recommend? Justify.   (2 marks)

....

....

Question 5.4

A 78-year-old Chinese man with a background of diabetes, hypertension, ischaemic heart disease and advanced dementia was admitted with a mechanical fall. He had a longstanding history of chronic alcoholism until his cognition and day-to-day functioning started deteriorating in recent months. His family was finding it difficult to care for him at home and after the necessary assessment, nursing home placement was planned. The extent of care was discussed with his family; in view of his advanced age and co-morbidities, it was decided that escalation of care was not appropriate in the event of deterioration and that he was unsuitable for intensive care unit (ICU) management or cardiopulmonary resuscitation.

At around 8 pm on the third day of admission, the night staff nurse found him to be drowsy and disorientated. He looked flushed and sweaty. His vital signs were: temperature 37.5°C, blood pressure 100/46 mmHg, pulse rate 110/min, respiratory rate 16/min and oxygen saturation 91% on room air. The house officer on call noted that the patient looked flushed and sweaty. His pupils were 5 mm bilaterally and reactive to light. The chest and neurological examinations were grossly unremarkable.

Routine blood tests were requested and he was started on intranasal oxygen 24% and normal saline infusion. On review in an hour, he was stuporous. His blood pressure was 70/30 mmHg and his pulse rate 140/min. Investigation results were:

Hb	12.5 g/dl	(12–16)
WBC Count	16.47 × 10(9) /L	(4–10)
Platelet	467 × 10(9) /L	(140–440)
Blood Urea	11.2 mmol/L	(2.7–6.9)
Sodium	132 mmol/L	(136–146)
Potassium	5.1 mmol/L	(3.5–5.1)
Bicarbonate	16.4 mmol/L	(19–29)
Chloride	93 mmol/L	(98–107)
Serum Creatinine	136 µmol/L	(45–84)
Glucose	8.9 mmol/L	(4.4–7.8)
Blood Ketone	0.0 mmol/L	(0.0–0.6)

ECG sinus tachycardia
Chest X-ray unremarkable

1.   Identify the biochemical syndrome.   (1 mark)

....

2.   Suggest three IMPORTANT tests that you would call the laboratory to urgently *add* to the above.   (3 marks)

a. ....

b. ....

c. ....

While waiting for the result, the nursing staff noted that the 500 mL bottle of alcohol-based hand rub (contains isopropyl alcohol 70%) at the bedside was uncovered and completely empty. A quick review of the closed-circuit TV footage showed that the patient had

consumed the entire bottle at around 7.30 pm. You remember that
isopropyl alcohol is primarily metabolised to acetone.

3. **Which of the following is the next MOST appropriate**
   course of management? (2 marks)

   a. Arrange for hospice care
   b. Discuss terminal discharge with family
   c. Provide best supportive care in the ward
   d. Transfer to ICU
   e. Transfer to nursing home ( )

While discussing with the consultant on call and his family, the
patient collapsed. He was expeditiously intubated and sent to the
ICU. His blood pressure remained low despite normal saline infusion, and he required inotropic support. His urine output remained
poor over the next six hours, with his hourly output dropping to
zero. Further investigations revealed the following:

Blood Urea	16.2 mmol/L	(2.7–6.9)
Sodium	142 mmol/L	(136–146)
Potassium	5.4 mmol/L	(3.5–5.1)
Bicarbonate	14.2 mmol/L	(19–29)
Chloride	95 mmol/L	(98–107)
Serum Creatinine	224 μmol/L	(45–84)
Glucose	13.2 mmol/L	(4.4–7.8)
Blood Ketone	1.6 mmol/L	(0.0–0.6)
Lactate	6.4 mmol/L	(0.5–2.2)
Serum Osmolality	374 mmol/kg	(275–301)

ABG result on 15L oxygen through non rebreathing mask prior to intubation:

pH	7.12	(7.37–7.45)
pCO_2	56 mmHg	(35–45)
pO_2	126 mmHg	(75–100)
Base Excess	11.2 mmol/L	(2.0–2.0)
Oxygen Saturation	96%	
Standard Bicarbonate	15.5 mmol/L	(21–27)

Urine microscopy no crystals

4A. Comment on the osmolal gap. (2 marks)

....

....

4B. Comment on the blood ketone level. (2 marks)

....

....

4C. Postulate two possible explanations for the high lactic acid level. (2 marks)

a. ....

b. ....

4D. Postulate two possible explanations for the high serum creatinine level. (2 marks)

a. ....

b. ....

4E. What is the significance of the urine microscopy result? (1 mark)

....

5. What does the blood gas analysis indicate? (2 marks)

....

Fomepizole, an inhibitor of alcohol dehydrogenase, is used in methanol or ethylene glycol poisoning to prevent the generation of toxic metabolites.

6. What is your thought about using this drug in this patient? (1 mark)

....

....

In spite of adequate hydration and inotropic support to maintain adequate blood pressure, he remained oligo-anuric.

7. **Which of the following is the next MOST appropriate step in management?** (2 marks)

    a. Continuous renal replacement therapy without need for frusemide
    b. Haemodialysis without need for frusemie
    c. Intravenous frusemide so that dialysis can be delayed
    d. Intravenous frusemide while dialysis is considered
    e. Listing for urgent renal transplantation.   (   )

Question 5.5

A 36-year-old female presented to the emergency department for swollen painful joints and fever of two weeks' duration. Five weeks ago, she underwent a dental procedure, after which flu-like symptoms developed. She was treated with antibiotics, and an extensive local search for complications of the procedure was negative.

In the course of the past two weeks, her fever reached a peak of 40°C in the evenings. She lost 5 kg in weight. There were no unusual symptoms localising to the gastrointestinal tract, urogenital tract or eyes.

1. **Based on the history alone, suggest two differential diagnoses.** (2 marks)

    a. ....

    b. ....

A physical examination showed an obviously sick woman. Her vital signs were: temperature 39.6°C, blood pressure 140/70 mmHg and pulse rate 96/min. An examination of her heart, lungs, abdomen, skin and eyes were all unremarkable. There were signs of mild inflammation (stress pain and joint-line tenderness) of the left wrist, left knee (plus small effusion) and right ankle. After specifically inspecting the patient during her fever in the evening a rash on the trunk was observed.

Below is her temperature chart:

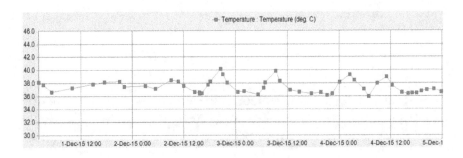

2A. Describe the pattern of fever observed.   (2 marks)

....

....

2B. Give two differential diagnoses for this pattern of fever in an adult.   (2 marks)

a. ....

b. ....

Below are her initial laboratory test results:

Full Blood Count			
Haemoglobin	10.6	⬇	[14.0-18.0 G/DL]
WBC Count	24.83	⬆	[4.0-10.0 X10(9)/L]
Platelet Count	589	⬆	[140-440 X10(9)/L]
RBC Count	3.75	⬇	[4.5-6.3 X10(12)/]
Haematocrit	32.1	⬇	[38-52 %]
MCV	85.6		[78-98 FL]
MCH	28.3		[27-32 PG]
MCHC	33.0		[32-36 G/DL]
RBC Distribution Width	14.5		[10.9-15.7 %]
Mean Platelet Volume	10.6		[7.2-11.1 FL]
....Differential Count*	********		
Neutrophil	93.3	⬆	[40-75 %]
Lymphocyte	4.0	⬇	[15-41 %]
Monocyte	0.7	⬇	[2-10 %]
Eosinophil	1.7		[0-6 %]
Basophil	0.3		[0-1 %]
Neut Absolute	23.18	⬆	[2.0-7.5 X10(9)/L]
Lymph Absolute	0.99	⬇	[1.0-3.0 X10(9)/L]
Mono Absolute	0.17	⬇	[0.2-0.8 X10(9)/L]
EOS Absolute	0.42		[0.04-0.44 X10(9)/L]
BAS Absolute	0.07		[0-0.1 X10(9)/L]

Renal Panel			
Urea, serum	3.9		[2.7-6.9 MMOL/L]
Sodium, serum	132	⬇	[136-146 MMOL/L]
Potassium, serum	4.3		[3.6-5.0 MMOL/L]
Chloride, serum	100		[100-107 MMOL/L]
Bicarbonate, serum	23.7		[19.0-29.0 MMOL/L]
Creatinine, serum	54		[54-101 UMOL/L]

Liver Panel			
Protein Total, serum	56	⬇	[68-85 g/L]
Albumin, serum	27	⬇	[40-51 g/L]
Bilirubin Total, serum	4	⬇	[7-32 umol/L]
Alkaline Phosphatase,	97		[39-99 U/L]
Alanine Transaminase,	115	⬆	[6-66 U/L]
Aspartate Transaminase,	165	⬆	[12-42 U/L]
Gamma-Glutamyl	78	⬆	[6-42 U/L]

Erythrocyte Sedimentation Rate (ESR)   113 ⬆[1–10 MM/HR]
C-Reactive Protein (CRP), serum   262 ⬆[0.2–9.1 MG/L]

3. **Fill in the box below with your interpretation of the respective abnormality *in this patient*. Row E has been completed for illustration.**   (1 × 4 = 4 marks)

A	Haemoglobin (her baseline haemoglobin checked before the dental procedure was 12.4 g/dL)	
B	White blood cell count	
C	Platelet count	
D	Liver enzymes	
E	Serum albumin	Low likely due to acute systemic inflammation

On admission, aerobic and anaerobic blood cultures were also performed. Her chest X-ray and urine microscopic examinations were normal. She was put on an intravenous broad-spectrum antibiotic. **At 48 hours, the blood cultures returned as negative.**

4. **Suggest four MOST appropriate investigations at this stage.**   (4 marks)

    a. ....

    b. ....

    c. ....

    d. ....

Results of extensive investigations were negative except for serum ferritin 14,262.0 ug/L (13.0–15.0). The patient was still febrile and unwell.

5. What is the MOST likely clinical diagnosis? (2 marks)

....

6. What is the MOST appropriate initial treatment for this problem? (2 marks)

....

Two days later, she became progressively unwell. These are her laboratory test results:

Full Blood Count			
Haemoglobin	6.9	⬇	[14.0-18.0 G/DL]
WBC Count	2.88	⬇	[4.0-10.0 X10(9)/L]
Platelet Count	60	⬇	[140-440 X10(9)/L]
RBC Count	2.21	⬇	[4.5-6.3 X10(12)/]
Haematocrit	19.5	⬇	[38-52 %]
MCV	88.2		[78-98 FL]
MCH	31.2		[27-32 PG]
MCHC	35.4		[32-36 G/DL]
RBC Distribution Width	14.1		[10.9-15.7 %]
Mean Platelet Volume	11.7	⬆	[7.2-11.1 FL]
....Differential Count*	********		
Neutrophil	95.0	⬆	[40-75 %]
Lymphocyte	4.0	⬇	[15-41 %]
Monocyte	0.0	⬇	[2-10 %]
Eosinophil	0.0		[0-6 %]
N. Myelocyte	1.0	⬆	[%]
Nucleated RBC	3/100 WBC		
Neut Absolute	2.73		[2.0-7.5 X10(9)/L]
Lymph Absolute	0.12	⬇	[1.0-3.0 X10(9)/L]
Mono Absolute	0.00	⬇	[0.2-0.8 X10(9)/L]
EOS Absolute	0.00	⬇	[0.04-0.44 X10(9)/L]
N.Myelocyte Abs	0.03		[X10(9)/L]

Liver Panel			
Albumin, serum	35	⬇	[40-51 G/L]
Bilirubin Total, serum	99	⬆	[7-32 UMOL/L]
Alkaline Phosphatase, serum	268	⬆	[39-99 U/L]
Alanine Transaminase, serum	2010	⬆⬆	[6-66 U/L]
Aspartate Transaminase, serum	4840	⬆⬆	[12-42 U/L]
Gamma-Glutamyl Transferase,	328	⬆	[14-94 U/L]

Coagulation Profile			
Prothrombin Time	14.7	⬆	[9.9-11.4 SECS]
APTT	62.0	⬆	[25.7-32.9 SECS]

Erythrocyte Sedimentation Rate (ESR) 5 [1-10 MM/HR]

7. **Suggest a possible explanation for the observed changes.**
    (1 mark)

    ....

8. **What is the MOST likely explanation for her low erythro-cyte sedimentation rate?**
    (1 mark)

    ....

Assessment Paper
6

Question 6.1

A 45-year-old female was rushed to the emergency department after receiving intramuscular diclofenac for her shoulder pain at her general practitioner's clinic. About 30 minutes later, she developed swelling in her face, lips and eyelids, and a rash. She felt weak and dizzy. She gave a history of taking diclofenac injection and tablets in the past without any reaction. She denied taking other drugs or being bitten by insects. Her vital signs were: temperature 36.8°C, pulse rate 104/min, regular, respiratory rate 24/min, 92% oxygen saturation on room air and blood pressure 92/52 mmHg. On examination, she had pronounced and uniform oedema affecting her eyelids, lips and cheeks.

1. **Which of the following physical examinations would be of crucial importance?** (2 marks)

    a. Cardiorespiratory auscultation
    b. Determination of the presence of collapsing pulse
    c. Determination of jugular venous pressure
    d. Determination of standing blood pressure
    e. Inspection of mucosal surfaces of anogenitalia (   )

2A. A skin examination of her upper chest revealed:

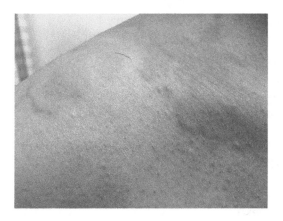

What is the most likely diagnosis?   (1 mark)

    a. Acute eczema
    b. Erythroderma (generalised exfoliative dermatitis)
    c. Fixed drug eruption (multifocal)
    d. Maculopapular exanthem
    e. Urticaria   (   )

2B. Skin examination of the leg revealed:

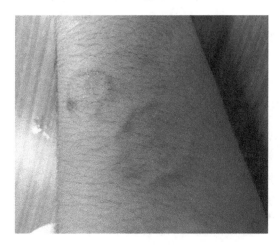

What is the most likely diagnosis?   (1 mark)

   a. Erythema chronicum migrans
   b. Erythema multiforme
   c. Insect bite reaction
   d. Tinea corporis
   e. Urticarial vasculitis   (   )

3A. Which of the following pharmacological interventions should be administered expeditiously?   (2 marks)

   a. Adrenaline
   b. Crystalloid
   c. Hydrocortisone
   e. Oxygen
   f. Promethazine   (   )

3B. Specify the dose and route.   (2 marks)

....

Five minutes later, the nurse reports the patient's vital signs as: pulse rate 110/min, regular, respiratory rate 26/min, 90% oxygen saturation on room air and blood pressure 90/45 mmHg. The patient is also wheezing.

4. Which of the following pharmacological interventions should be immediate upon this evaluation?   (2 marks)

   a. Adrenaline
   b. Crystalloid
   c. Hydrocortisone
   d. Oxygen
   e. Promethazine   (   )

5.   Which of the following blood tests is diagnostic?

(2 marks)

    a.   Absolute eosinophil count
    b.   Erythrocyte sedimentation rate
    c.   Serum histamine level
    d.   Serum tryptase level
    e.   Total immunoglobulin E level   (   )

6.   Select TWO from the list of options, which are risk multipliers for a severe reaction.

(2 marks)

    a.   Age
    b.   Gender
    c.   History of asthma
    d.   History of atopic eczema
    e.   Recent ingestion of traditional Chinese medicine
    f.   Recent ingestion of calcium
        channel blockers   (   ) & (   )

The patient responds to treatment, and her vital signs normalise over the next ten minutes.

7.   What is the next MOST appropriate plan of action?

(2 marks)

    a.   Admit for overnight observation
    b.   Discharge right away with a course of oral antihistamines
    c.   Keep in the emergency department for one hour before discharging her
    d.   Set up an intravenous cannula and infuse fluids over 24 hours
    e.   Set up an intravenous cannula and infuse diphenhydramine

(   )

8. **What else will you do for the patient before she goes home?**
                                                              (4 marks)

    ....

    ....

    ....

    ....

Question 6.2

A 25-year-old migrant (Southeast Asian) worker presented with a severe headache, fever and vomiting. His symptoms started a day ago and did not resolve with paracetamol, prompting his dormitory co-inhabitants to bring him to the emergency department. On arrival, his vital signs were: temperature 38.2°C, blood pressure 100/60 mmHg and heart rate 110/min. His Glasgow Coma Scale (GCS) was E4V5M6. His tongue was dry, and he looked lethargic. His heart, lung and abdominal examinations were unremarkable. There was a faint but not blanchable rash on his lower limbs that was not noticed in the morning by the patient. There was neck stiffness.

1. **Fill in the box below to indicate a clinical assessment on the head and neck that should be performed and its purpose. The first row has been completed for illustration purposes.** (4 marks)

	Physical examination on head and neck (1 × 2 = 2 marks)	Purpose (1 × 2 = 2 marks)
A	Facial tenderness	Screen for underlying sinusitis, which could have a nidus for intracranial infection.
B		
C		

The additional physical examination was unremarkable.

2.   What is the MOST likely clinical diagnosis?   (1 mark)

....

3.   Name two MOST likely aetiological agents in each of these groups.   (2 × 2 = 4 marks)

A. Bacterial:
a. *Neisseria meningitidis*

b. ....

c. ....

B. Non-bacterial:
a. ....

b. ....

Treatment, including an intravenous drug, was given in the emergency department, and he was quickly admitted only after a full blood count and renal panel. Upon admission, he mentioned that this had happened twice before.

4.   Apart from instituting early antibiotics, give three other key initial management principles for this patient.   (3 marks)

a. ....

b. ....

c. ....

5. **List four specific pharmacologic therapies (doses not required) that should be administered to this patient.**
    (4 marks)

    a. ....

    b. ....

    c. ....

    d. ....

You subsequently received reports of his previous two similar episodes and the laboratory report of this episode. All three episodes were caused by meningococcus.

6. **What specific public health measure should be instituted as soon as possible?** (2 marks)

    ....

7. **What further investigations should be performed for this patient?** (2 marks)

    ....

    ....

Question 6.3

A 43-year-old banker presented to the emergency department for a shortness of breath of two days. He was a non-smoker with a medical history of hyperlipidaemia. He had travelled to Penang, Malaysia, on a bus a few days ago.

On arrival, his vital signs were: temperature 36.6°C, blood pressure 139/83 mmHg, pulse rate 97/min, respiratory rate 23/min and oxygen saturation 92% on room air.

His chest X-ray and electrocardiogram are shown below.

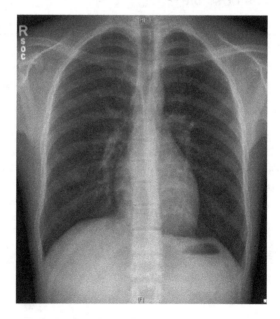

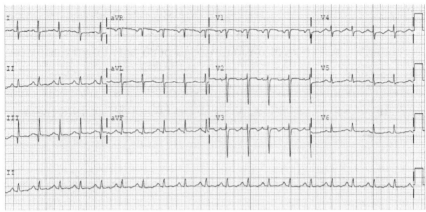

1. **Identify the abnormalities from these preliminary investigations.** (2 marks)

   a. ....

   b. ....

2. **Give two MOST likely differential diagnoses.** (2 marks)

   a. ....

   b. ....

During a physical examination, the patient fell unconscious and became unresponsive. He was cold and clammy to the touch, and his pulse was not palpable. His stat electrocardiogram essentially showed the same features as above.

3. **Name the present clinical syndrome.** (1 mark)

   ....

Cardiopulmonary resuscitation (CPR) immediately commenced. After five minutes of CPR, the patient had a return of spontaneous circulation. Endotracheal intubation had been performed during the resuscitation.

His vital signs were: blood pressure 60/40 mmHg, pulse rate 120/min and oxygen saturation 98% on FiO_2 100% on mechanical ventilation.

4.   What is the next MOST important intervention? (1 mark)

....

5.   Which of the following *diagnostic* investigations should be urgently performed upon haemodynamic stability?
                                                                (2 marks)

    A. CT brain scan
    B. CT pulmonary angiogram
    C. Arterial blood gas
    D. Transthoracic echocardiogram
        a. A and C only
        b. B and D only
        c. A, B and C
        d. B, C and D
        e. D only   (   )

6.   However, if the patient remains haemodynamically unstable, which of the above diagnostic investigations should still be urgently performed?   (2 marks)

    a. A only
    b. B only
    c. C only
    d. D only
    e. None of the above   (   )

The patient subsequently stabilised with a blood pressure reading of 120/70 mmHg and pulse rate of 110/min. He remained intubated and ventilated using assisted control/ventilator control (ACVC) mode ventilation, positive end-expiratory pressure (PEEP) 5 mmHg, FiO_2 40% and tidal volume 500 ml.

His arterial blood gas showed pH 7.48, pCO_2 30 mmHg, pO_2 75 mmHg, HCO_3 20 mEq/L and SaO_2 92%.

7. What is your interpretation of these results? (2 marks)

....

....

8. What is the next MOST appropriate intervention?
(1 mark)

....

The patient was discharged after a 3-day stay in the intensive care unit and a 1-week stay in the ward. However, he returned a month later to the emergency department with blood in his vomitus. You went through his medication list and found out that he had been discharged with warfarin.

Preliminary investigations showed a haemoglobin level of 7.8 g/dL (12–16) and an international normalised ratio (INR) of 10.

9. List four urgent therapeutic interventions. (4 marks)

a. ....

b. ....

c. ....

d. ....

After the bleeding was arrested and the patient stabilised, a decision was made to re-initiate warfarinisation. He was also prescribed omeprazole regularly until an outpatient review.

10. What advice concerning therapeutics would you give him?   **(3 marks)**

....

....

....

Question 6.4

A 78-year-old lady visited the outpatient clinic after having had a fall at home. Her past medical history comprised of poorly controlled chronic obstructive pulmonary disease (on multiple inhalers and requiring one to two hospital admissions per year), type 2 diabetes mellitus (latest HbA1c 10.4%), ischaemic heart disease and rheumatoid arthritis.

Her daughter was very concerned about her mother as this was her second fall in three months. The patient claimed that she felt more "clumsy" of late and on a few occasions, also felt light-headed. She has been independent in her activities of daily living and ambulation, but since the most recent fall, she has been needing supervision.

1. **Based on this clinical history, suggest four MOST likely reasons for her falls.** (4 marks)

   a. ....

   b. ....

   c. ....

   d. ....

In view of her recurrent falls, some blood tests were ordered and their results are as follow:

Haemoglobin	9.8 g/dL	(12–16)
WBC Count	8.17 × 10(9)/L	(4–10)
Platelet Count	179 × 10(9)/L	(140–440)

Blood Urea	7.2 mmol/L	(2.7–6.9)
Sodium	123 mmol/L	(136–146)
Potassium	5.0 mmol/L	(3.5–5.1)
Bicarbonate	18.7 mmol/L	(19–29)
Chloride	106 mmol/L	(98–107)
Serum Creatinine	102 µmol/L	(44–80)
Glucose	13.3 mmol/L	(3.9–11)
Urine Spot Sodium	32 mmol/L	

2A. Give two MOST likely explanations for her sodium level. She is clinically euvolaemic.   (2 marks)

a. ....

b. ....

2B. Suggest two MOST appropriate follow-on investigations.
(2 marks)

a. ....

b. ....

As part of the evaluation of her bone health, a bone mineral density scan (BMD) was ordered:

	BMD (g/cm²)	T-score
Lumbar Spine	0.537	–4.1
Femoral Neck	0.434	–3.5
Total Hip	0.385	–4.6

3A. What is the diagnosis? (1 mark)

....

3B. For this diagnosis, identify four risk factors in this patient based on the available history above. (4 marks)

a. ....

b. ....

c. ....

d. ....

3C. Name an assessment scale that will help you evaluate her long-term fracture risk. (1 mark)

....

The daughter said that she has been coaxing her mother to drink one full glass of cow's milk daily to improve calcium intake.

4.   Which of the following advice is the MOST appropriate for her? (1 mark)

a. Continue the same and encourage sun exposure
b. Convert one glass of cow's milk to one glass of soya bean milk daily and encourage sun exposure
c. Convert one glass of cow's milk to two glasses of soya bean milk daily and encourage sun exposure
d. Drink two glasses of cow's milk daily and encourage sun exposure
e. Needs calcium and Vitamin D supplements   (   )

5.   In addition to your advice, which of the following medication is the MOST appropriate? (1 mark)

a. Bisphosphonate
b. Calcitonin
c. Cox-2 inhibitor
d. Magnesium
e. Oestrogen-progestin   (   )

This is a picture of the patient's hands.

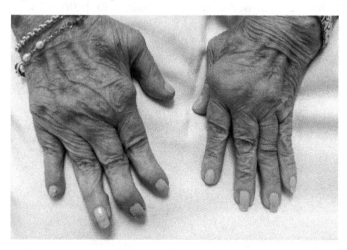

6. **What is the anatomical pathology that explains the swelling of the metacarpophalangeal joints?** (1 mark)

....

7. **Suggest three MOST likely explanations of her low haemoglobin level in relation to this condition.** (3 marks)

a. ....

b. ....

c. ....

Question 6.5

An 18-year-old Chinese male presented to the clinic with a lack of pubertal development.

1. **What is the value of obtaining a family history of a similar complaint?** (1 mark)

    ....

    ....

This male had no significant family or past medical history of note. He had centripetal obesity with bilateral gynaecomastia. He was tall (1.75 m) with a eunuchoid habitus. His testicles were small and firm (3 ml volume each).

2. **What is the value in examining the olfactory and optic nerves?** (2 marks)

    ....

3. **What is the clinical significance of a tall stature in this patient with delayed puberty as opposed to another patient with short stature and delayed puberty?** (2 marks)

    ....

    ....

Detailed examination revealed normal cranial nerves.

4.   **What is the MOST likely clinical diagnosis?**   (1 mark)

....

5.   **What other supporting physical findings would you look for?**   (2 marks)

....

....

Further investigations revealed FSH 0.2IU/L (1.5–12.4), LH undetectable and testosterone 1.4 nmol/L (10.3–31).

6.   **Which of the following is the next MOST appropriate investigation?**   (2 marks)

    a. Chromosomal analysis on peripheral blood lymphocytes to specifically look for 47,XXY karyotype
    b. Chromosomal analysis on peripheral blood lymphocytes to specifically look for 47,XYY karyotype
    c. Urinary gonadotropin assay to specifically look for abnormal levels
    d. MRI hypothalamus-pituitary to specifically look for structural abnormalities or tumours
    e. Testicular biopsy to specifically look for Leydig cell atrophy   (   )

He was given depot intramuscular testosterone in graduated doses and showed good clinical improvement with a gradual development of secondary sexual characteristics. Over the years he was maintained on testosterone injections at 3-week intervals.

7. What would you monitor biochemically at regular intervals besides his clinical responsiveness? (2 marks)

....

....

During one of the clinics visits many years after initiating regular testosterone injections, the following laboratory results were noted:

Haemoglobin	18.6 g/dL	(13.0–17.0)
Haematocrit	54.1%	(42–52)
Red Blood Cells	6.25 × 10(9)/L	(4.5–6.3)
WBC Count	9.35 × 10(9)/L	(4–10)
Platelet Count	201 × 10(9)/L	(140–440)
MCV	75.7 fL	(78.0–98.0)
MCH	22.2 pg	(27.0–32.0)
MCHC	29.3 g/dL	(32.0–36.0)
RBC Distribution Width	16.7%	(10.9–15.7)

8. Fill in the box with specific areas in history that you would ask and why. (2 marks)

	History	Purpose/Significance
a.		
b.		

Clinically, he appeared plethoric. Conjunctivae were injected, and his tongue was purplish. Few scratch marks were noted on the limbs.

9. **Fill in the box with other specific physical findings that you would look for and why.** (2 marks)

	Physical finding	Purpose/Significance
a.		.
b.		

The rest of the examination was unremarkable. He appeared otherwise well.

10. **Give two relevant investigations that you would order.** (2 marks)

    a. ....

    b. ....

He declined all further evaluation or referrals. The below graphs depict the trend of his haemoglobin and haematocrit depicted over the years.

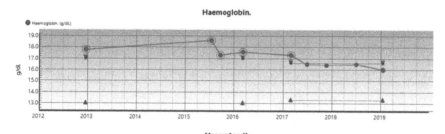

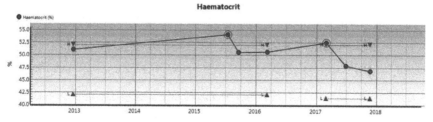

11. **Postulate two explanations for the lowering of his haemoglobin and haematocrit levels.** (2 marks)

a. ....

b. ....

Assessment Paper
7

Question 7.1

A 68-year-old woman presented to the emergency department with a 1-month history of shortness of breath on exertion and leg swelling. A review of her systems was negative for chest pain, palpitations and syncope. She had a background of hypertension of six years for which she had been taking amlodipine 10 mg OM and hydrochlorothiazide 25 mg OM. She had no history of myocardial infarction. Two days prior, she had seen her general practitioner who changed her hydrochlorothiazide to frusemide 40 mg OM.

Her vital signs were blood pressure 180/90 mmHg, pulse rate 82/min regular, oxygen saturation 96% on 4L oxygen. Her BMI was 30 kg/m². A physical examination revealed increased jugular venous distension. Chest auscultation revealed bilateral crepitations at lung bases but no cardiac murmurs. Her liver was not palpable. Pitting oedema was present to the mid-shin level.

1. **Suggest two MOST likely causes for her clinical presentation.** (2 marks)

   a. ....

   b. ....

2. **Which of the following is the MOST appropriate initial management?** (2 marks)

    a. Administer oral aspirin 300 mg
    b. Administer glyceryl trinitrate patch
    c. Intravenous frusemide 40 mg
    d. Intravenous labetolol 20 mg
    e. Transthoracic echocardiogram to help determine
       next step   ( )

This is her electrocardiogram:

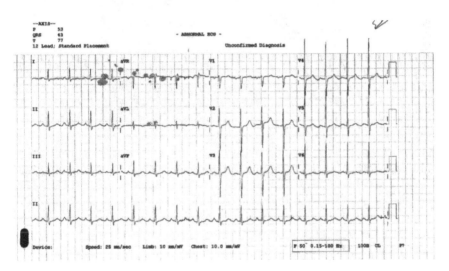

3. **Identify two electrocardiographic abnormalities.**
                                                      (2 marks)

    a. ....

    b. ....

This is her chest X-ray:

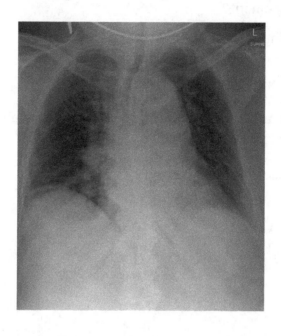

4.   Identify two radiographic abnormalities.   (2 marks)

a. ....

b. ....

5.   Suggest six other MOST relevant blood investigations that you would order at this stage.   (0.5 x 6 = 3 marks)

a. ....

b. ....

c. ....

d. ....

e. ....

f. ....

A Doppler transthoracic echocardiography showed moderate concentric left ventricular hypertrophy, no significant valvular abnormalities, no pericardial effusion and no regional wall abnormalities. Her left ventricular ejection fraction was 60%.

6.   Summarise and justify the MOST likely clinical diagnosis.
                                                            (3 marks)

....

....

....

7.   Which of the following is the MOST important outcome to aim for in the management of this condition?   (1 mark)

a. Improvement in her exercise capacity
b. Improvement in her symptoms and health-related quality of life
c. Reduction in all-cause mortality
d. Reduction in mortality from cardiovascular disease
e. Reduction in recurrent hospital admission with heart failure   (   )

8.   Which of the following is the MOST appropriate therapy to optimise the control of her blood pressure?   (2 marks)

a. Add bisoprolol
b. Add hydralazine
c. Add prazosin
d. Add losartan
e. Double the dose of amlodipine   (   )

After an uneventful stay in the hospital, the patient was discharged with frusemide, amlodipine, perindopril and atorvastatin. She was given an outpatient review in a month.

On the morning of the review, she complained of a burning sensation in her mouth. She recalled she ate boiled bird's nest — for the first time in her life — after dinner the evening before.

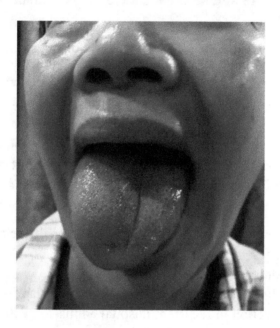

9.   What is the MOST appropriate management?   (2 marks)

    a. Endotracheal intubation

    b. Expectant management (observation)

    c. Intramuscular promethazine

    d. Intramuscular triamcinolone

    e. Subcutaneous adrenaline   (   )

10. **What is the MOST appropriate advice?** (1 mark)

a. Avoid bird's nest in future
b. Referral to allergist for skin prick testing, KIV re-challenge
c. Replace frusemide with hydrochlorothiazide/ spironolactone
d. Stop all medications until reviewed by allergist
e. Stop perindopril ( )

Question 7.2

A 70-year-old man, a chronic smoker of 50 pack-years with no known medical history of note, complained of worsening shortness of breath over the last six months. He was prescribed with a salbutamol inhaler by his general practitioner but with minimal symptom relief. He was referred to your clinic for further management.

1. **Based on his history alone, suggest three MOST likely differential diagnoses for his shortness of breath.**
    (3 marks)

    a. ....

    b. ....

    c. ....

On examination, he was afebrile, blood pressure 140/80 mmHg, heart rate 90/min and respiratory rate 20/min. His oxygen saturation was 98% on ambient air. His heart sounds were dual, with no murmurs heard. Auscultation of his lungs revealed no adventitious sounds.

His chest radiograph was as shown:

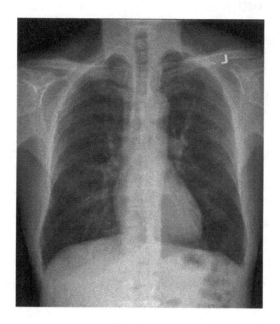

Spirometry was also performed:

	Pred	LLN	Actual	%Pred
---- SPIROMETRY ----				
FEV1 (L)	2.12	1.21	1.16	55
FVC (L)	3.12	1.90	2.99	96
FEV1/FVC (%)	79	71	39	49

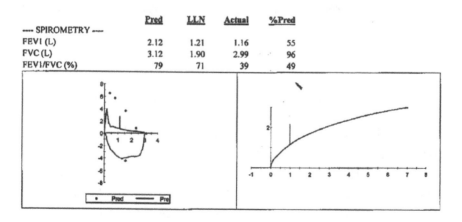

2.   What is your clinical diagnosis based on the investigations? Justify.   **(3 marks)**

....

....

....

3.   Suggest two other appropriate INITIAL investigations.
                                                                            (2 marks)

a. Arterial blood gas
b. 12-lead ECG
c. Coronary angiogram
d. CT thorax
e. Diffusing capacity of lung for carbon monoxide
f. Full blood count
g. Transthoracic echocardiography   (   ) & (   )

4.   Outline three key management principles.   **(3 marks)**

a. ....

b. ....

c. ....

Two months later, this patient complained of a sudden onset of chest pain and severe shortness of breath. At the emergency department, he was disorientated but still able to follow instructions. His temperature was 36.9°C, blood pressure 188/93 mmHg, pulse rate 120/min, respiration rate 32/min and oxygen saturation 83% on room air. He was obviously using his accessory muscles of breathing. His jugular venous pressure was normal. Auscultation of lungs revealed decreased breath sounds with polyphonic end-expiratory wheezing throughout both lung fields. No peripheral oedema was noted.

5. **Suggest three MOST urgent considerations of his acute presentation.** (3 marks)

   a. ....

   b. ....

   c. ....

6. **What is the MOST appropriate next step in his management?** (1 mark)

   a. Immediately intubate the patient
   b. Immediately provide oxygen via a Venturi mask
   c. Immediately provide oxygen via a non-rebreather mask
   d. Order an antihypertensive drug stat
   e. Perform arterial blood gas before starting any form of oxygen therapy ( )

His arterial blood gas revealed:

pH	7.317
$PaCO_2$	62.2 mmHg
PaO_2	75 mmHg
Bicarbonate	26.1 mmol/L
SaO_2	92.5%

7. **What is your interpretation of the blood gas result?**
                                                    (1 mark)

    ....

8. **Outline three key management principles.**   (3 marks)

    a. ....

    b. ....

    c. ....

9. **Is this patient particularly prone to developing osteo-
    porosis?**   (1 mark)

    ....

Question 7.3

A 78-year-old lady with a history of glaucoma, hypertension and diabetes mellitus was brought to the emergency department because of increasingly frequent visual hallucinations. Specifically, she described seeing "little women dressed in ancient costumes". She was not frightened and even attempted to have conversations with them. Her daughter also observed that the patient had become increasingly forgetful over the last one year.

1. Based on this history alone, give four MOST likely differential diagnoses for the presentation at the emergency department. (4 marks)

   a. ....

   b. ....

   c. ....

   d. ....

2. Fill in the box below with four specific areas in the history that would be relevant to arriving at the differential diagnoses, and the respective significance.
(1 x 4 = 4 marks)

	Aspect of history to take	**Significance**
A		
B		
C		
D		

On examination, she appeared well-hydrated and comfortable. She was afebrile, had a regular pulse with rate of 84/min, and blood pressure of 150/70 mmHg. She had a slight resting tremor in both hands. Apart from mild cogwheel rigidity, no other neurological findings were elicited. The rest of the systemic examination was unremarkable.

3. What is the MOST important step to complete the examination at this juncture?
(2 marks)

....

Her full blood count, renal panel, electrolytes, thyroid function and Vitamin B12 level returned as unremarkable. A computed tomography of the head showed only age-related cerebral involution.

4.   **What is the MOST likely diagnosis and give the MOST likely aetiology?**   (2 marks)

Diagnosis: ....

Aetiology: ....

Upon admission, the patient was placed on fall precautions.

5.   **What are her risk factors for falls?**   (3 marks)

....

....

6.   **What nursing orders on monitoring *pertaining to her acute presentation* would you request for upon the patient's admission?**   (2 marks)

....

....

The ward team decided to start her on pharmacological treatment.

7.   **What is your treatment of choice for her cognition and visual hallucinations?**   (1 mark)

....

8.   **Name one class of medication that should be avoided in this patient. Justify.**   (2 marks)

....

....

Question 7.4

A 43-year-old man presented with a fever of four days' duration. He had a past history of hypertension and paraplegia after a road traffic accident six years ago. He has a long-term indwelling urinary catheter, which was last changed a week ago. His fasting blood glucose level was 4.4 mmol/L at his last screening in a polyclinic.

Upon physical examination, his temperature was 38.4°C, blood pressure 135/90 mmHg and pulse rate 84/min. He weighed 70 kg. His neurological examination was notable for flaccid paraplegia with sensorimotor loss below T6 level. No abnormality was found in the cardiovascular, respiratory and abdominal systems. The urine collected from his urinary catheter looked cloudy.

An examination of his right foot showed the following:

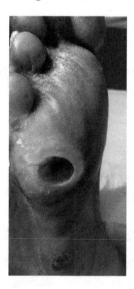

1A. What is the MOST likely aetiology of this ulcer? Justify.
                                                              (3 marks)

....

....

1B. Suggest an appropriate wound dressing.   (1 mark)

....

**1C. Apart from wound dressings, give two management prin-
       ciples for this ulcer.   (2 marks)**

   a. ....

   b. ....

A urine Dipstix showed the following:

Glucose	Trace
Ketones	Negative
Blood	1+
Protein	1+
Bilirubin	Negative
Nitrite	Negative
Leucocytes	3+

**2.   Given the clinical scenario so far, what is the MOST likely
       cause of the fever?   (1 mark)**

....

The patient was admitted for a workup. His blood culture grew *Klebsiella pneumoniae*. A contrast-enhanced CT scan of his abdomen/pelvis was performed.

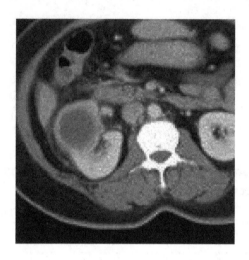

3.   What is the clinico-radiological diagnosis?   (2 marks)

....

The patient was started on intravenous gentamicin of 4 mg/kg q24H. After a week of treatment, his urine output was noted to increase to over 5 litres per day. His renal panel showed the following:

Blood Urea	6 mmol/L	(4.7–6.9)
Sodium	146 mmol/L	(135–145)
Potassium	2.9 mmol/L	(3.5–5)
Bicarbonate	18 mmol/L	(22–26)
Chloride	130 mmol/L	(95–105)
Serum Creatinine	95 µmol/L	(70–100)
Calcium	2.30 mmol/L	(2.1–2.45)
Magnesium	0.91 mmol/L	(0.74–0.97)

4. Which of the following is the next MOST appropriate investigation? (2 marks)

a. Arterial pH
b. Plasma osmolality
c. Urine osmolality
d. Urine pH
e. Urine potassium ( )

5. What is his estimated water deficit? (2 marks)

a. 2 litres
b. 3 litres
c. 4 litres
d. 5 litres
e. Not enough data to estimate ( )

A water deprivation test was administered.

Time (h)	0800	0900	1000*	1100	1200
Urine osmolality (mOsm/kg)	175	180	190	195	205
Plasma osmolality (mOsm/kg)			298		

5 units of aqueous vasopressin was given at 1000 h

6. What is your interpretation of the test results? (2 marks)

....

....

7.   What is the MOST likely cause of this abnormality?
                                                              (1 mark)

....

The patient eventually recovered and was discharged after one week. When the home nurse reviewed the patient in three months to change the urinary catheter, she noted that the urine appeared concentrated. The patient was otherwise well. She performed a urine Dipstix that showed:

Glucose	Trace
Ketones	Negative
Blood	Negative
Protein	1+
Bilirubin	Negative
Nitrite	Negative
Leucocytes	2+

8.   Which of the following should be the MOST appropriate action by the home nurse?   **(2 marks)**

a. Direct patient to the emergency department for admission for parenteral antibiotic
b. Inform a doctor to prescribe an empirical course of amoxicillin-clavulanate
c. Inform a doctor to prescribe an empirical course of levofloxacin
d. Change the urinary catheter and discard urine
e. Change the urinary catheter and send urine for culture

                                                              (   )

9. **Suppose the patient undergoes a water deprivation test now, which of the following graphs will MOST likely be observed?** (2 marks)

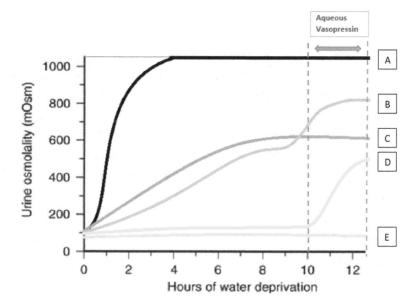

Question 7.5

A 65-year-old lady self-palpated a lump in her left breast. A mammogram showed features that highly suggested breast cancer. She underwent a lumpectomy and sentinel lymph node dissection. Histopathology showed a 1.3 cm grade 2 infiltrative ductal carcinoma with oestrogen/progesterone receptor positivity, and Her-2 overexpression. The sentinel lymph node was negative for malignancy. On review in the clinic, there was no visible or palpable recurrence in the left breast.

1. **Give four clinical signs that you would look for in this patient.** (4 marks)

   a. ....

   b. ....

   c. ....

   d. ....

2. **Which of the following is the next MOST appropriate step?** (2 marks)

   a. Proceed to complete mastectomy and axillary clearance
   b. Request for CT chest, abdomen and pelvis
   c. Request for ultrasound pelvis
   d. Send blood for BRCA1 and BRCA2 genetic mutations
   e. Start adjuvant chemotherapy ( )

She declined adjuvant cytotoxic chemotherapy because of potential cardiotoxicity.

3. Which of the following is the MOST appropriate management? (2 marks)

a. Close monitoring with regular 6-monthly scans
b. Leuprorelin (gonadotrophin-releasing hormone agonist)
c. Ovarian ablation by surgery or radiation
d. Tamoxifen (E2 receptor blocker)
e. Trastuzumab (monoclonal humanised IgG1 that targets human epidermal growth factor receptor HER-2)   (   )

She declined all interventions and defaulted on her follow-up. One year later, she complained of lethargy, anorexia and significant weight loss over 2 months.

4. Which of the following is the MOST important blood test to order? (2 marks)

a. Blood culture
b. CA 15-3
c. Calcium
d. CEA
e. Procalcitonin   (   )

Subsequent investigations revealed metastases in her mediastinal lymph nodes, internal mammary lymph node, and multiple vertebrae. In particular, she had been developing increasing back pain.

5. List three symptoms that could suggest metastatic cord compression. (3 marks)

a. ....

b. ....

c. ....

These symptoms were absent, and she had no clinical signs of cord compression. She adamantly refused cytotoxic chemotherapy.

6.   Which of the following is the MOST appropriate treatment?
                                                    (2 marks)

   a. Bisphosphonate
   b. Dexamethasone
   c. Leuprorelin (gonadotrophin-releasing hormone agonist)
   d. Radiotherapy
   e. Tamoxifen   (   )

The patient still had severe back pain despite taking paracetamol 1 g QDS. The pain was constant and aching, localised to her mid-thoracic spine region with no radiation. Her renal and liver function tests were normal.

7.   Which of the following is the NEXT most appropriate pharmacological management?   **(2 marks)**

   a. Calcitonin
   b. Gabapentin
   c. Non-steroidal anti-inflammatory drug
   d. Morphine
   e. Tramadol   (   )

With the therapy, her baseline pain was better controlled, but she still complained of a sharp stabbing pain that was worse on movement. Results of electrodiagnostic testing were in keeping with neuropathic pain. Adjuvant analgesia was considered.

8. **Which of the following is the MOST appropriate initial drug to provide adjuvant analgesia for this lady?**

(1 mark)

 a. Oral codeine
 b. Etoricoxib
 c. Lignocaine patch
 d. Intramuscular pethidine
 e. Pregabalin   ( )

Shortly after starting this medicine, she developed a painful rash over her left arm.

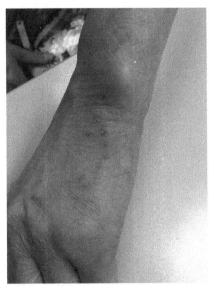 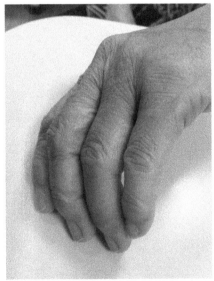

9. **What is the MOST likely diagnosis?**   (2 marks)

....

Assessment Paper

8

Question 8.1

A 65-year-old man presented with fever, chills and flank pain. He was found to have right pyelonephritis. His past medical history was notable for nasopharyngeal carcinoma ten years ago, which was successfully treated with radiation therapy.

Here are the blood culture and sensitivity results:

Organism: *Escherichia coli*

Ampicillin	R
Amoxicillin/Clavulanate	S
Piperacillin/Tazobactam	S
Cefazolin	S
Ceftriaxone	S
Cefepime	S
Aztreonam	S
Amikacin	S
Gentamicin	R
Ciprofloxacin	R
Trimethoprim/Sulfamethoxazole	R
Fosfomycin	S
Nitrofurantoin	S

1A. What is the single MOST appropriate treatment?

(2 marks)

....

1B. **What is the single MOST appropriate drug if he has a history of penicillin allergy?** (1 mark)

....

2. **What total duration of antibiotic should be considered for him?** (1 mark)

....

Since admission, he was found to have persistent hyponatraemia (sodium between 126 and 129 mmol/L) though he was clinically euvolaemic. The following tests were then ordered:

Free T4	9.1 pmol/L	(12.7–20.3)
Thyroid-stimulating Hormone	0.292 mIU/L	(0.701–4.280)
8 am Cortisol	305 nmol/L	(123–626)

3A. **What is your interpretation of the thyroid function test?** (1 mark)

....

3B. **Give two MOST likely causes of it.** (2 marks)

a. ....

b. ....

4. **What is your interpretation of the cortisol result?** (2 marks)

....

....

5. **What aspects of history and/or physical examination would you perform in the evaluation of this patient? Do not give specific details but give your answer in groupings. An example has been provided as an illustration.**
(6 marks)

a. Manifestations (or symptoms and signs) of hypothyroidism

b. ....

c. ....

d. ....

e. ....

f. ....

g. ....

The ward team plans to start him on thyroxine replacement.

6. **What investigation should be performed *before* starting thyroxine replacement? Explain your rationale.** (2 marks)

....

....

By the fifth day of admission, the fever has lysed, but the patient developed non-bloody diarrhea, about eight times for the past two days.

7. **What is the MOST appropriate investigation?** (1 mark)

....

8. **What is the MOST appropriate intervention?** (2 marks)

....

Question 8.2

A 45-year-old lady complained of an acute onset of severe abdominal pain, nausea and vomiting. Her pain was worst over the epigastric region, sharp in nature and lasted several hours. The pain did not radiate, and no specific aggravating or relieving factors were noted. There were no infective symptoms. She had been constitutionally well with no change in bowel habits.

Past medical history includes hypertension on amlodipine 5 mg OM and diabetes on metformin 500 mg BD. Her most recent HbA1c was 9%. She has had no surgery before.

On examination, she was diaphoretic and afebrile. Her vital signs were blood pressure 90/50 mmHg, heart rate 110/min, respiratory rate 26/min and oxygen saturation 94% on room air. Her body mass index (BMI) was 35 kg/m^2. Her heart sounds were dual, and breath sounds were vesicular. An abdominal examination revealed diffuse tenderness with rebound and guarding over her epigastric region. Bowel sounds were sluggish.

1. **Suggest four MOST likely differential diagnoses.**

(4 marks)

a. ....

b. ....

c. ....

d. ....

Primary investigations showed the following:

Haemoglobin	11 g/dL	(12–16)
Haematocrit	48%	(38–52)
White Cell Count	15 × 10(9)/L	(4–10)
Platelet	117 × 10(9)/L	(140–400)
Blood Urea	10 mmol/L	(4.7–6.9)
Sodium	150 mmol/L	(135–145)
Potassium	4.5 mmol/L	(3.5–4.5)
Bicarbonate	13 mmol/L	(19–29)
Chloride	90 mmol/L	(98–107)
Serum Creatinine	180 μmol	(60–90)
Bilirubin	38 mmol/L	(7–32)
Aspartate Transaminase	200 U/L	(6–66)
Alanine Transaminase	227 U/L	(12–42)
Alkaline Phosphatase	300 U/L	(39–99)
Albumin	30 mmol/L	(40–51)
Lactate	5.0 mmol/L	(0–1.9)
Calcium	2.03 mmol/L	(2.1–2.45)
Glucose	23 mmol/L	(4–8)
Amylase	1100 mmol/L	(4–300)
Total Cholesterol	9.8 mmol/L	(<5.2)
Triglycerides	16 mmol/L	(1.7–2.2)
LDL-cholesterol	unmeasurable	
Arterial pH	7.23	(7.35–7.45)
PaO_2	80 mmHg	(70–100)
$PaCO_2$	30 mmHg	(35–45)

The doctor also sent her blood for a coagulation profile and group and cross-match in case urgent surgery was necessary.

2. **Suggest four other MOST urgent investigations (excluding abdominal imaging) that should have been performed at the start.** (4 marks)

   a ....

   b. ....

   c. ....

   d. ....

3. **In the light of the above biochemical findings, what specific physical findings would you examine for in this patient?** (2 marks)

   ....

   ....

4. **Give the complete diagnosis for this patient.** (2 marks)

   ....

   ....

5. **Give two aspects of history that you would take in regard to clarifying the aetiology of this acute presentation.** (2 marks)

   a. ....

   b. ....

6. What are the next MOST appropriate management steps to take? Indicate Yes or No for each of these recommendations. (4 marks)

A. Abdominal X-ray   (   )
B. Admission to intensive care unit   (   )
C. Aggressive fluid resuscitation   (   )
D. Allowance of enteral feeding   (   )
E. Broad-spectrum antibiotics   (   )
F. CT scan of the abdomen and pelvis   (   )
G. Endoscopic retrograde cholangiopancreatography (   )
H. Intravenous insulin   (   )

The patient made good recovery after one week of monitoring and treatment. However, she complained of these painful lesions on her legs.

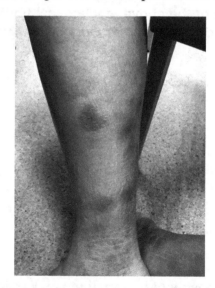

A skin biopsy was performed.

7. Predict the histological abnormalities observed. (2 marks)

....

....

Question 8.3

A 60-year-old man presented with a cough of three months' duration. He has been smoking 20 sticks of cigarettes per day for the past 40 years. He also reported intermittent haemoptysis, and hoarseness of voice.

1. **How does each of the following aspects help you narrow your differential diagnoses?**

   A. That the duration of symptoms is three months instead of three days? (1 mark)

   ....

   B. That the haemoptysis occurred after coughing instead of after physical exertion? (1 mark)

   ....

   C. That the cough had no predilection for time of the day instead of it being nocturnal? (1 mark)

   ....

2. **Give three MOST likely differential diagnoses based on this history alone.** (3 marks)

   a. ....

   b. ....

   c. ....

A physical examination showed partial right eyelid ptosis and the following:

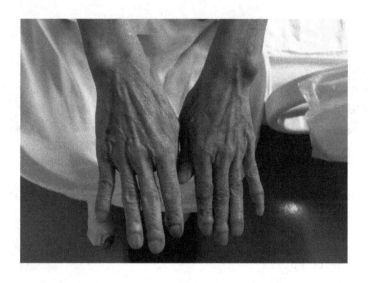

3A. Identify the abnormality/abnormalities shown in the picture above.   (1 mark)

....

3B. What other clinical signs on his face would you look for?
(2 marks)

....

....

His chest radiograph is shown as below:

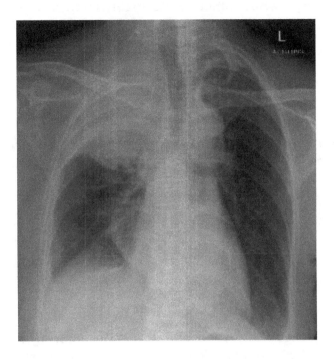

4. Which of the following clinical signs in the respiratory system would MOST likely be present in this patient?

(1 mark)

a. Absent breath sounds on the right upper chest
b. Aegophony on the right upper back
c. Asymmetrical chest expansion on the back
d. Bronchial breath sounds on the right upper chest
e. Dullness to percussion on the right upper back   (   )

5. **Study the chest X-ray carefully. Apart from the apical opacity, what other abnormality/abnormalities is/are present?**   (2 marks)

....

....

6. **Suggest two MOST likely causes for his hoarseness of voice.**   (2 marks)

a. ....

....

b. ....

....

7. **Rank the following investigations in order of highest to lowest diagnostic yield for the above clinical problem.**   (2 marks)

   a. Bronchoscopy
   b. Pan-CT (brain, thorax, abdomen)
   c. Spirometry
   d. Sputum cytology
   e. Sputum for acid-fast bacilli PCR
      and culture   (   ) > (   ) > (   ) > (   ) > (   )

After running through some investigations, the pathologist read a tissue sample taken from the lesion.

8. **Which of the following is the MOST likely histological diagnosis in this patient?** (1 mark)

   a. Carcinoid tumour
   b. Non-Hodgkin lymphoma
   c. Non-small cell lung carcinoma
   d. Small cell lung carcinoma
   e. Tuberculosis   (   )

The patient declined all treatments and discharged himself against medical advice. A month later, he was re-admitted for breathlessness. When you saw him in the morning rounds, he was sitting up and breathing heavily. His face was oedematous with a purplish hue. He said he had not slept the whole night as he could not lie down flat.

9. **Explain why he is orthopnoeic.** (1 mark)

   ....

10. **What is the MOST appropriate treatment plan?** (2 marks)

   1. Chemotherapy and/or radiotherapy
   2. Intravenous glucocorticoids
   3. Intravenous thrombolysis
   4. Low-molecular-weight heparin
   5. 4-drug anti-tuberculosis regime
      a. (1) only
      b. (1) + (2)
      c. (3) + (4)
      d. (2) + (3) + (4)
      e. (5) only   (   )

Question 8.4

A 40-year-old pub singer was brought to the emergency department after his wife noticed that he was agitated and confused. He had been complaining of dyspnoea, fever and lethargy over the past four days.

On arrival, his vital signs were temperature 38.7°C, blood pressure 180/132 mm Hg, pulse rate 110/min and oxygen saturation of 80% on room air.

Supplemental oxygen was given and arterial blood gas was performed:

pH	7.204	(7.35–7.45)
pCO_2	87.7 mmHg	(35–45)
pO_2	72.3 mmHg	(75–100)
Base excess	3.5 mmol/L	(−2.0–2.0)
SpO_2	91.2%	(95–100)
HCO_3	26.2 mmol/L	(21–27)

1. **What is the biochemical syndrome?**   (2 marks)

    ....

This was the electrocardiogram:

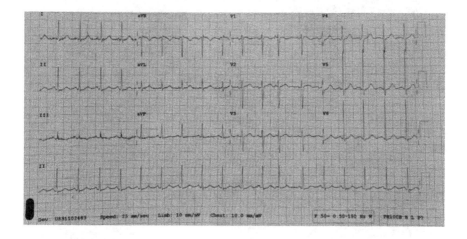

2.   Identify two electrocardiographic abnormalities.

(2 marks)

a. ....

b. ....

In view of the respiratory distress, he was immediately intubated and sent to the intensive care unit. On clinical examination, it was discovered that his jugular venous pressure was raised. His palms were sweaty, and he was tremulous. Auscultation of his lungs revealed bilateral crepitations. He had sacral and scrotal oedema. On closer examination of his legs, some firm lesions were noticed.

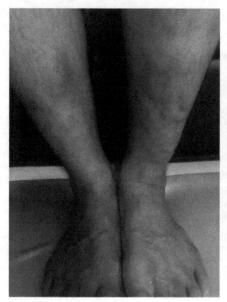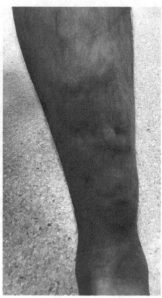

3A. **Describe the morphology of the skin lesions.**   (2 marks)

....

3B. **What is the chemical nature of the skin deposit?** (1 mark)

....

3C. **Where else would you look for similar lesions in the patient?**   (1 mark)

....

His initial blood test results showed:

Sodium	129 mmol/L	(136–146)
Potassium	3.9 mmol/L	(3.5–5.1)
Chloride	101 mmol/L	(98–107)
Bicarbonate	28 mmol/L	(19–29)
Creatinine	49 μmol/L	(45–84)

A bedside cardiac echocardiogram revealed an ejection fraction of 25%, moderate mitral regurgitation and regional wall abnormality.

4.   What is the MOST likely explanation for the hyponatraemia?
(1 mark)

....

5.   What is the MOST appropriate way to correct the hyponatraemia in this patient?   (2 marks)

....

6.   Which of the following classes of medication has been shown to improve the survival rate in a person similarly presenting with heart failure? Select three.   (3 marks)

a. Alpha-1 blocker
b. Angiotensin system blocker
c. Beta blocker
d. Calcium channel blocker
e. Cardiac glycoside
f. Centrally-acting blocker
g. Mineralocorticoid receptor antagonist
h. Thiazide diuretic   (   ) & (   ) & (   )

7. **Given the patient's clinical features and findings so far, what is the MOST likely clinical syndrome at presentation?** (1 mark)

....

The appropriate treatment was instituted, and this patient's symptoms improved. He was subsequently discharged home on medical treatment. Four months later, after he had achieved good hormonal control, he underwent surgery to remove the entire organ responsible for his symptoms.

8. **What is the MOST important surgical risk that this patient should be warned about?** (1 mark)

....

On the first post-operative day, he complained of perioral numbness and tingling of his fingers.

9. **What is the MOST likely explanation for these new symptoms?** (2 marks)

....

....

10. **Give two clinical signs that you might elicit.** (2 marks)

    a. ....

    b. ....

Question 8.5

A 55-year-old nurse with well-controlled mild hypertension pre-sented with lower limb swelling, which gets particularly worse after prolonged standing at work, for a few years. She also complained of having ankle pains at times during prolonged standing. She took an occasional diuretic to improve the swelling. Other than some generalised aches and pains that were attributed to osteoarthritis, she was well. Her weight has remained stable at 72 kg for her height of 1.6 m.

1. **Given this clinical presentation, which of the following are plausible causes for her lower limb swelling? Select two.** (2 marks)

    a. Addison's disease
    b. Constrictive pericarditis
    c. Pelvic malignancy
    d. Rapidly progressive glomerulonephritis
    e. Rheumatoid arthritis
    f. Systemic lupus erythematosus   (   ) & (   )

2. **What is the significance of each of the following addi-tional history?** (2 marks)

    A. Lower limb swelling worse before her periods

    ....

    B. Chronic diarrhea

    ....

A drug history revealed that her symptoms worsened after being switched to amlodipine therapy.

3.   Which of the following drugs are also well known causes of lower limb oedema? Select two.   (2 marks)

    a. Bisoprolol
    b. Doxycycline
    c. Etoricoxib
    d. Gliclazide
    e. Lisinopril
    f. Prednisolone   (   ) & (   )

While she accepted that the oedema was a side-effect of amlodipine and was willing to live with it, she was worried that she had seen patients presenting with oedema who turned up having more serious conditions. She was particularly concerned as she recalled that the oedema was mild even before the introduction of amlodipine. She had no arthritis and had a recent electrocardiogram and chest X-ray (routine screening), which were both normal.

    Initial relevant investigations are as follow:

Hb	11.5 g/dl	(12–16)
WBC Count	8.26 × 10(9)	(4–10)
Platelet	259 × 10(9)	(140–440)
MCV	90 fL	(78–98)
ESR	127 mm/hr	(1–10)
Serum Creatinine*	97 μmol/L	(45–84)
Serum Protein	99 g/L	(63–83)
Serum Albumin	37 g/L	(35–50)
Serum ALP	50 U/L	(39–99)
Serum ALT	12 U/L	(6–66)
Serum AST	12 U/L	(12–42)

TSH	1.520 mIU/L	(0.27–4.200)
Free T4	15.3 pmol/L	(11.8–24.6)
Urine alb:cr Ratio	0.6 mg/mmol	(0–3.5)

* It was noted that her serum creatinine was trending upwards gradually from 76 µmol/L when previous records were checked.

4A.   Comment on the serum protein level.   (2 marks)

....

....

4B.   What is the MOST likely clinical diagnosis? Justify.
(4 marks)

....

....

....

5.   Give two further important investigations.   (2 marks)

a. ....

b. ....

Urine protein electrophoresis showed elevated lambda free chains of 338 mg/L (5.7–26.3).

6A.   In the light of this finding, explain why the urine albumin-creatinine ratio was normal.   (1 mark)

....

6B.   What is/are the renal risk(s) associated with these light chains?   (2 marks)

....

....

7A.   What is the next MOST appropriate diagnostic investigation?
(1 mark)

....

7B.   What finding(s) would you expect from this investigation?
(1 mark)

....

In the past week, she had a skull X-ray performed when she complained of a headache.

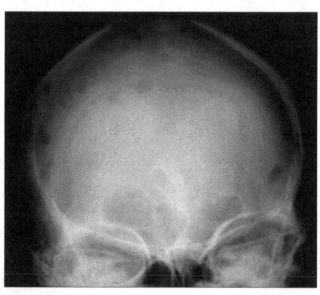

8.   What is your radiological interpretation?   (1 mark)

....

Assessment Paper

9

Question 9.1

A 25-year-old teacher presented with severe low back pain after carrying heavy books. An X-ray confirmed an L1 vertebral fracture. As the bones showed generalised translucency, the doctor further ordered bone mineral densitometry. The radiographer enquired about her last menstrual period, which she said occurred two weeks ago.

Here are her bone mineral density results:

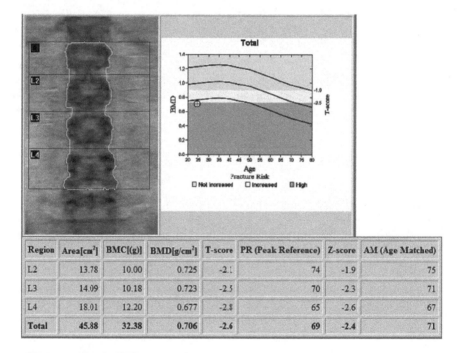

Region	Area[cm²]	BMC[(g)]	BMD[g/cm²]	T-score	PR (Peak Reference)	Z-score	AM (Age Matched)
L2	13.78	10.00	0.725	-2.1	74	-1.9	75
L3	14.09	10.18	0.723	-2.3	70	-2.3	71
L4	18.01	12.20	0.677	-2.8	65	-2.6	67
Total	45.88	32.38	0.706	-2.6	69	-2.4	71

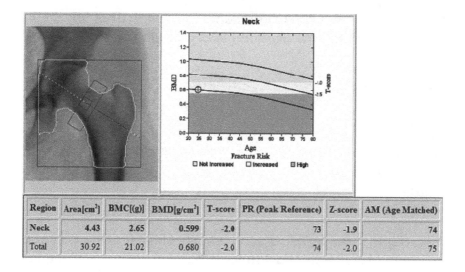

Region	Area[cm²]	BMC[(g)]	BMD[g/cm²]	T-score	PR (Peak Reference)	Z-score	AM (Age Matched)
Neck	4.43	2.65	0.599	-2.0	73	-1.9	74
Total	30.92	21.02	0.680	-2.0	74	-2.0	75

1. **Which of the following is the MOST appropriate interpretation?**

    (2 marks)

    a. Low bone density by Z-score classification
    b. Normal bone density by T-score classification
    c. Normal bone density by Z-score classification
    d. Osteopenia by Z-score classification
    e. Osteoporosis by T-score classification   ( )

On further history-taking, she revealed that she had been diagnosed with hypertension since her pregnancy five years ago. Her blood pressure had been well controlled with amlodipine 5 mg OM. She neither smoked nor drank alcohol. However, she noticed a gradual increase in weight since her pregnancy, from 70 kg to 100 kg, despite exercising and controlling her diet.

2.   Based on the clinical presentation so far, what important aspect of her medication history would you ask?

(1 mark)

....

....

A clinical examination revealed a truncally obese woman with puffy cheeks and facial hair. Her blood pressure reading was 160/95 mmHg.

3.   Name three MOST discriminatory clinical signs that you would make an effort to look for.   (3 marks)

a. ....

b. ....

c. ....

A hormonal workup was performed:

Test	Result	Reference Range
8 am Cortisol after an overnight 1 mg dexamethasone dose	337 nmol/L	<140 nmol/L
24-hr urinary free cortisol (1st sample) Urine volume: 1,200 ml	100 nmol/day	59–413 nmol/day
24-hr urinary free cortisol (2nd sample) Urine volume: 2,000 ml	152 nmol/day	
Adrenocorticotropic hormone (ACTH)	2.7 ng/L	10–60 ng/L

4A. What is the diagnosis?   (2 marks)

....

4B. What is your interpretation of the urinary free cortisol?
                                                   (1 mark)

....

....

A CT scan of her abdomen was performed, and an abnormality is
marked with an arrow.

5.   What anatomy does the lesion arise from?   (2 marks)

....

6.   What treatment option should be offered to this patient?
                                                   (1 mark)

....

7. **Prior to the treatment option offered to the patient, which of the following considerations is appropriate? Indicate (A) for appropriate and (I) for inappropriate.**   (3 marks)

a. Fine-needle biopsy of the lesion to exclude malignancy   (   )
b. Screen for diabetes mellitus and optimise glycemic control   (   )
c. Adequate cover with intravenous steroids during and after the treatment   (   )

Blood and urine investigations were also performed on the same day:

Sodium	140 mmol/L	(136–146)
Potassium	3.4 mmol/L	(3.5–5.1)
Bicarbonate	30 mmol/L	(19–29)
Creatinine	63 µmol/L	(44–80)
Magnesium	0.7 mmol/L	(0.74–0.97)
Calcium (corrected)	2.4 mmol/L	(2.1–2.6)
Urine potassium, 24-hr	35 mmol/day	(4–42)

8. **What are your interpretations of and conclusions drawn from these results?**   (3 marks)

    ....

    ....

    ....

    ....

9. **Summarise the pathophysiologic basis for the potassium result.** (2 marks)

....

....

....

....

Question 9.2

An 80-year old lady was referred by the nursing home for increasingly poor oral intake. She has a history of Alzheimer's disease, atrial fibrillation, hypertension, type 2 diabetes mellitus, osteoporosis and bilateral knee osteoarthritis. Her medications included risperidone 1 mg ON, digoxin 125 mcg OM, enalapril 5 mg BD, bisoprolol 2.5 mg OM, metformin 850 mg BD, glipizide 5 mg BD, and alendronate 70 mg, once weekly.

1. **Given this limited history, suggest four likely causes for her presentation that are:**

    A. Related to the gastrointestinal tract.   (2 marks)

    a. ....

    b. ....

    B. Not related to the gastrointestinal tract.   (2 marks)

    a. ....

    b. ....

On clinical examination, she was dehydrated and drowsy. Her vital signs showed: temperature 36.0°C, blood pressure 100/60 mmHg, pulse rate 75/min and oxygen saturation 94% on room air. The nurse from the home remarked that although the patient's overall oral intake was poor, they successfully fed her all usual medications.

2.   What immediate bedside test should be performed?
(1 mark)

....

Her electrocardiogram (ECG) is shown below.

Image courtesy of Dr Seow Swee Chong

3.   Identify two electrocardiographic abnormalities.
(2 marks)

a. ....

b. ....

4.   What is the MOST likely clinical diagnosis?   (2 marks)

....

Further investigations revealed:

Haemoglobin   11 g/dL   (12–16)
White Cell Count $15.42 \times 10(9)$/L   (4–10)

Platelet	$280 \times 10(9)$/L	(140–400)
Blood Urea	11.5 mmol/L	(4.7–6.9)
Sodium	128 mmol/L	(135–145)
Potassium	3.0 mmol/L	(3.5–4.5)
Chloride	160 mmol/L	(98–107)
Serum Creatinine	180 μmol/L	(60–90)

Chest X-ray: Right lower zone infiltrates
CT Brain: Age-related generalised involution. No acute infarct or intracranial haemorrhage.

5.   Give three immediate management principles. (3 marks)

a. ....

b. ....

c. ....

The next morning, she appeared more alert. Her caregiver tried to feed her breakfast. Drooling and coughing were noted as the patient was being fed. A resting tremor was also evident in her right hand.

6.   What is the clinical significance of the patient's reaction to the feeding? (1 mark)

....

7.   Suggest two MOST likely causes for this reaction.
(2 marks)

a. ....

b. ....

During her admission, the patient was placed on a modified diet with nectar-thickened fluids as recommended by the speech therapist. Her oral intake remained suboptimal, with less than half share taken at meal times. She complained of central chest discomfort, but a serial ECG and cardiac enzymes did not suggest acute coronary syndrome.

8. What is the MOST likely cause of the chest discomfort *in this patient*? (2 marks)

....

Her concerned daughter enquired about further management for her persistent poor intake.

9. Select three MOST appropriate management steps. (3 marks)

   a. Discourage dietary restriction of low sodium and diabetic diet
   b. Encourage daughter to bring her favourite food
   c. Refer to dietician
   d. Refer to psychiatrist
   e. Start oral mirtazapine
   f. Switch risperidone to quetiapine
   g. Trial of nasogastric tube feeding (   ) & (   ) & (   )

Question 9.3

1. **In each of these characteristics of diplopia obtained from history-taking, identify the lesion.** (2 marks)

    A. Diplopia resolved with head tilting to the side of the normal eye.

    ....

    B. Diplopia resolved with head rotation to the side of the affected eye.

    ....

2. **For each of these characteristics or situations of diplopia, provide one clinical example.** (3 marks)

    A. Intermittent diplopia

    ....

    B. Diplopia with ataxia

    ....

    C. Diplopia with contralateral hemiplegia

    ....

This is how the patient looked like at first glance:

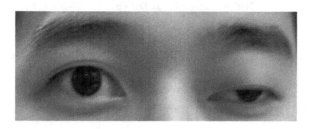

3. In the context of the left ptosis, provide one clinical example for each of the following additional physical finding. (3 marks)

A. Small left pupil

....

B. Large left pupil

....

C. The abnormality is overcome on an upward gaze

....

The patient's appearance, as shown above, was when he was asked to look forward in a resting position.

4. What is the MOST likely diagnosis? Explain. (2 marks)

....

....

5.   Based on the diagnosis, what is the clinical significance of each of these additional physical findings? (2 marks)

A. Left pupil was dilated and non-reactive to light

....

B. Left pupil was normal and reactive to light

....

Lateral eye movements were tested.

Asked to look right   Asked to look left

6.   What additional information can you draw from these observations? (2 marks)

....

....

7.   Suggest one possible diagnosis for each of these situations. (2 marks)

A. With pain in the eyes

....

B. Without pain in the eyes

....

The visual fields of this man are shown on formal perimetry below.

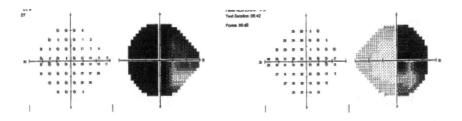

8. **Describe the visual field abnormality.** (2 marks)

....

9. **What is the unifying diagnosis for this patient?** (2 marks)

....

Question 9.4

A 58-year-old man with diabetes, hypertension, ischaemic heart disease and progressive chronic kidney disease (CKD) who had defaulted on previous renal clinic appointments presented with uraemic symptoms, fluid overload and progression of his CKD to end-stage.

1. **Give two cutaneous signs of uraemia that may be observed in this man.** (2 marks)

    a. ....

    b. ....

He was initiated on dialysis through a right internal jugular tunneled dialysis catheter. As required by national guidelines, his Hepatitis B, C and HIV serologies were requested prior to the initiation of dialysis:

Hepatitis B Surface Antigen (HBsAg)	Negative	
Hepatitis B Surface Antibody (Anti-HBs)	<2 IU/L	
Hepatitis B Core (HBC) Total Antibody	Reactive	
Hepatitis C Antibody Screen	Non-reactive	
HIV Screen	Non-reactive	
Serum Alanine Transaminase	12 U/L	(6–66)
Serum Aspartate Transaminase	31 U/L	(12–42)

2A. Interpret the results of the Hepatitis B serologies.
(3 marks)

....

....

....

....

2B. In the light of these results, what is the next MOST important blood test to perform? (1 mark)

....

He underwent a left radiocephalic arteriovenous fistula (AVF) creation and was discharged with the plan for haemodialysis thrice a week at a centre near his house. Three weeks after discharge, he developed fever and chills while undergoing dialysis and was readmitted to the hospital. He had some dry cough and no other symptoms. His vital signs were temperature 39°C, heart rate 100/min, blood pressure 100/66 mmHg, respiratory rate 18/min and oxygen saturation 99% on room air. A chest examination was unremarkable, and the recently created AVF was neither red nor tender. His blood results were as follow:

Hb	14.5 g/dL	(12–16)
WBC Count	$16.47 \times 10(9)$/L	(4–10)
Platelet	$178 \times 10(9)$	(140–440)
Blood Urea	23.5 mmol/L	(2.7–6.9)
Sodium	136 mmol/L	(136–146)
Potassium	5.7 mmol/L	(3.5–5.1)
Bicarbonate	16.8 mmol/L	(19–29)

Chloride	93 mmol/L	(98–107)
Serum Creatinine	668 umol/L	(45–84)
CRP	86 mg/L	(0.2–9.1)
Serum Procalcitonin	8.79 mcg/L	(< 0.49)
Troponin T	218 ng/L	(≤ 19)

ECG: sinus tachycardia
Chest X-ray: unremarkable

3.   **Which of the following is the MOST likely cause of his febrile illness?**   (1 mark)

a. AVF infection
b. Bacterial pneumonia
c. Catheter-related infection
d. Reactivation of viral hepatitis
e. SARS-COVID 19   (   )

4.   **What is the next MOST appropriate investigation?**
                                                              (1 mark)

....

5.   **What is the MOST common pathogen responsible for his febrile illness?**   (1 mark)

....

Below is his blood culture and sensitivity result.

ORGANISM: Methicillin-resistant *Staphylococcus aureus* (MRSA)

Penicillin	R
Ampicillin	R
Cloxacillin	R
Cefazolin	R
Gentamicin	S
Cotrimoxazole	S
Clindamycin	R
Vancomycin	S

6.   Which of the following is the MOST appropriate management?   **(2 marks)**

a. Catheter guidewire exchange + IV vancomycin
b. Catheter removal + IV vancomycin
c. IV vancomycin only
d. Vancomycin antibiotic lock + PO cotrimoxazole
e. None of the above   (   )

7.   Which of the following is the MOST appropriate end-point of treatment?   **(1 mark)**

a. Clearance of metabolic acidosis
b. Complete lysis of fever
c. Negative repeat blood cultures
d. Normal white blood cell count
e. Serum procalcitonin <0.49 mcg/L   (   )

Despite the appropriate intervention, he continued to be febrile after 96 hours, and repeated blood cultures continued to be positive for MRSA. His repeat blood results were as follow:

Hb	12.5 g/dL	(12–16)
WBC Count	19.58 × 10(9)/L	(4–10)
Platelet	64 × 10(9)	(140–440)
PT	14.6 sec	(9.9–11.4)
APTT	48 sec	(25.7–32.9)
Blood Urea	32.5 mmol/L	(2.7–6.9)
Sodium	136 mmol/L	(136–146)
Potassium	4.4 mmol/L	(3.5–5.1)
Bicarbonate	20.8 mmol/L	(19–29)
Chloride	107 mmol/L	(98–107)
Serum Creatinine	1068 μmol/L	(45–84)
CRP	321 mg/L	(0.2–9.1)
Serum Procalcitonin	87.49 mcg/L	(< 0.49)

8. **Suggest three MOST plausible reasons for the ongoing sepsis.**   (3 marks)

a. ....

b. ....

c. ....

9. **Suggest two MOST plausible reasons for the thrombocytopenia.** (2 marks)

    a. ....

    b. ....

During the morning round, the team doctor detected a cardiac murmur, which was previously absent. It was a grade 2/6 ejection systolic murmur heard all over the precordium but loudest over the mitral area.

10. **Give two MOST likely differential diagnoses.** (2 marks)

    a. ....

    b. ....

An urgent transthoracic echocardiography failed to reveal an abnormality.

11. **What is the next MOST appropriate investigation?** (1 mark)

....

Question 9.5

A 34-year-old man, with no medical history of note, presented with a 5-month history of low back pain. He reported stiffness in the mornings, which gradually improved by the afternoon. There was no history of trauma. He also admitted to having pain below his left heel for the last few months. A year earlier, he suffered a self-limiting episode of pain in the left shoulder and swelling in the right knee. He denied any skin, bladder or bowel problems. There was no relevant family history.

1. **Give four other aspects of history specifically directed at *aetiology* that you would like to ask.** (4 marks)

    a. ....

    b. ....

    c. ....

    d. ....

On examination, the only abnormal finding was a slight restriction of lateral lumbar flexion. A plain radiograph of his pelvis was reported as normal.

2. **What physical examination test would you perform to assess the forward flexion of the lumbar spine?** (1 mark)

    ....

3. **What are the MOST appropriate diagnostic investigations at this stage?** (3 marks)

....

....

....

4. **For each of the following interventions, state whether it is appropriate (A) or inappropriate (I) at this stage.**
(1 x 4 = 4 marks)

A. Bed rest for three weeks, and to resume work gradually

( )

B. Local injection of corticosteroid into tender point on heel

( )

C. Oral indomethacin ( )

D. Physiotherapy ( )

After a period of intervention, the patient achieved excellent pain relief of his low back pain and heel pain. He did not return for a subsequent review in the outpatient clinic.

Six years later, he was brought to the emergency department after his wife witnessed him fainting in the living room. He had regained consciousness after a few minutes but looked diaphoretic and unwell. He reported feeling unwell with a fever, sore throat and body ache for the past few days.

This is his electrocardiogram performed on arrival at the emergency department:

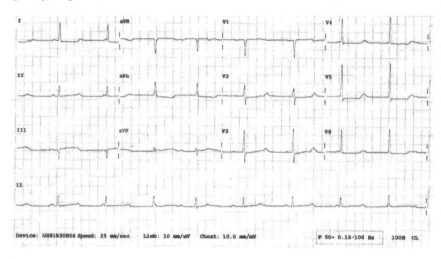

5A. Identify the key abnormalities. (2 marks)

....

....

5B. What is the diagnosis? (1 mark)

....

6. Suggest two MOST likely causes of this problem.
(2 marks)

a. ....

b. ....

A few hours later, his pulse rate dropped to 30/min. His blood pressure was 85/50 mmHg and oxygen saturation was 91% on room air. He also started complaining of chest pain and breathlessness.

7. What is the MOST appropriate immediate management?
(1 mark)

   a. Intramuscular adrenaline
   b. Intravenous atropine
   c. Intravenous dopamine
   d. Oxygen by non-rebreather mask
   e. Prepare for endotracheal intubation   ( )

When the patient was stabilised, it was concluded that this cardiac problem would most likely be permanent.

8. What is the MOST appropriate intervention to recommend?
(1 mark)

....

As part of cardiac evaluation, a transthoracic echocardiography was performed.

9. What primary structural abnormality might MOST likely be found?
(1 mark)

....

Assessment Paper

10

Question 10.1

A 44-year-old lady with type 2 diabetes diagnosed two years ago was brought to the hospital when her family found her unconscious. According to her husband, she had been having fever and multiple episodes of vomiting for five days. Her usual medications were gliclazide modified release (MR) 30 mg OM, sitagliptin 100 mg OM and metformin 500 mg BD.

At the emergency department, her vital signs were: temperature 38.2°C, heart rate 133/min, respiratory rate 40/min, blood pressure 78/52 mmHg and oxygen saturation 100% on room air. Her Glasgow Coma Score (GCS) was 7 (E4V1M2). She was noted to be cold and clammy. Her mucous membranes were dry. The general survey was otherwise unremarkable. Her capillary blood glucose was 2.2 mmol/L.

1. **Other than the low blood sugar, suggest two other possible causes of her low GCS score.** (2 marks)

   a. ....

   b. ....

2. **Which of the following is the MOST appropriate management of her sugar level?** (2 marks)

   a. Intramuscular glucagon 1 mg
   b. Intravenous dextrose 50% in 40 ml rapid bolus
   c. Intravenous dextrose 10% in 500 ml fast infusion

   d. Intravenous dextrose/saline in 500 ml fast infusion

   e. Nasogastric intubation for delivery of concentrated
     dextrose   (   )

3.   List two other management priorities.   (2 marks)

   a. ....

   b. ....

Fifteen minutes later, the lady remained stuporous. Her capillary blood glucose was 2.8 mmol/L.

4.   Which of the following is the next MOST appropriate management?   (2 marks)

   a. Intramuscular glucagon 1 mg

   b. Intravenous dextrose 50% in 40 ml rapid bolus

   c. Intravenous dextrose 10% in 500 ml fast infusion

   d. Intravenous dextrose/saline in 500 ml fast infusion

   e. Nasogastric intubation for delivery of concentrated
     dextrose   (   )

On re-assessment half an hour later, the patient regained consciousness. Her vital signs were: heart rate 128/min, respiratory rate 32/min, blood pressure 121/76 mmHg and oxygen saturation 100% on room air.

   The renal panel showed the following:

Blood urea	23.8 mmol/L	(4.7–6.9)
Sodium	132 mmol/L	(135–145)
Potassium	3.8 mmol/L	(3.5–4.5)
Bicarbonate	5.0 mmol/L	(19–29)

Chloride   95 mmol/L   (98–107)
Serum Creatinine   165 μmol/L   (60–90)

5A. Identify the MOST significant biochemical syndrome.

(2 marks)

....

5B. Suggest two MOST likely causes of this syndrome.

(2 marks)

a. ....

b. ....

5C. Outline three treatment principles for this syndrome in this patient.   (3 marks)

a. ....

b. ....

c. ....

After resolution of her acute illness, her medications were resumed.

6.   Which of the following is the MOST appropriate advice to her concerning medications, should she falls sick in the future and her blood sugar goes low?   (2 marks)

a. Omit glicazide MR
b. Omit metformin
c. Omit sitagliptin
d. Stop all diabetic medication
e. Continue all usual medication   (   )

She also asked about these itchy lesions on her limbs of six months' duration.

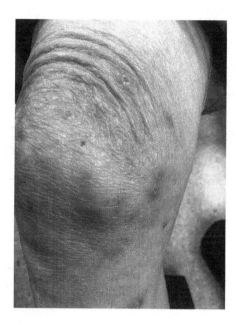

7.   Give two differential diagnoses.   (2 marks)

a. ....

b. ....

8.   Which of the following is the MOST appropriate initial treatment for these lesions?   (1 mark)

a. Betamethasone valerate 0.1% ointment
b. Hydrocortisone 1% cream
c. Intralesional triamcinolone acetonide 0.1%
d. Oral hydroxyzine
e. Oral prednisolone   (   )

Question 10.2

An 18-year-old man serving his National Service presented with a feeling of bloating, especially after food. He also complained of generalised lethargy and had been struggling to keep up with his squad members. His appetite was poor due to the bloating sensation and his mouth ulcers. He gave a history of weight loss over a year. Further, he observed he passed more frequent loose stool and intermittently felt feverish.

On examination, he was noted to be thin. Multiple oral ulcers were present. His abdomen was soft and distended with active bowel sounds on auscultation.

1A. **What is the MOST likely *underlying* clinical syndrome?**

(1 mark)

....

1B. **What would be an important differential diagnosis, supposing the patient told you he had been engaging in unprotected sexual intercourse with multiple partners?**

(2 marks)

....

2. In view of the clinical presentation above:

A. What nail changes would you look for?   (2 marks)

....

....

B. What findings would you look for in a rectal examination?
(2 marks)

....

....

Below are his abdominal X-rays:

3. Identify two radiographic abnormalities.   (2 marks)

a. ....

b. ....

4.   List three MOST appropriate stool investigations.

(3 marks)

a. ....

b. ....

c. ....

This is the sigmoid colon on colonoscopy:

5.   Describe two colonoscopic abnormalities.   (2 marks)

a. ....

b. ....

6.   Which of the following are appropriate differential diagnoses for these colonoscopic findings? Select three.

(3 marks)

a. Adenomatous polyposis coli

b. Amoebic dysentery

c. Candida colitis

d. Chronic diverticulitis

   e. Ischaemic colitis

   f. Lymphoma

   g. Sigmoid cancer

   h. Ulcerative colitis   (   ) & (   ) & (   )

A diagnostic biopsy showed features compatible with Crohn's disease, and the patient was commenced on systemic therapy. He maintained that there was absolutely compliance to the medication. Two weeks later, he was re-admitted for fever. His blood count showed pancytopenia.

7. Suggest two likely explanations for this occurrence.

                                                    (2 marks)

   a. ....

   b. ....

8. What pharmacotherapy may be useful to improve the white cell count?   (1 mark)

   ....

Question 10.3

A 44-year-old female with a past medical history of dyslipidaemia presented to the emergency department (ED) with a new onset seizure. She was cooking at that time and felt sudden weakness and numbness over her left upper and lower limbs. She subsequently became unconscious. Her husband witnessed repetitive jerking of all four limbs just prior to losing consciousness.

On arrival at the ED, she was conscious and orientated. She denied having a fever, headache or vomiting prior to the seizure. Her vital signs were: temperature 36.7°C, heart rate 119/min and blood pressure 138/84 mmHg.

1. **What would you ask the husband to lend further evidence of the occurrence of a seizure rather than a faint? Give two questions.** (2 marks)

    a. ....

    b. ....

2. **What questions on *social history or habits* would you ask the patient to look for a possible cause of the seizure? Give two.** (2 marks)

    a. ....

    b. ....

Her full blood count, renal function and liver function were unremarkable.

3. **Give three other initial investigations that you would do.**
(3 marks)

a. ....

b. ....

c. ....

The results of the investigations were normal. After discussing the risks and benefits of anti-epileptic therapy, she was very keen to prevent a recurrence. You intend to start her on sodium valproate.

4. **List two side-effects that you would warn her about.**
(2 marks)

a. ....

b. ....

5. **She works as a Grab (a ride-hailing app) driver. What advice would you give?** **(2 marks)**

....

....

Six months later, she re-presented to the ED with another seizure that was similar to her first.

6.   Give two evaluation principles.   (2 marks)

a. ....

b. ....

An MRI brain scan showed three cortical enhancing lesions with vasogenic oedema and mild mass effect in both frontal lobes including the precentral gyri.

T_1 T_2

7.   Give two differential diagnoses of the cortical lesions for each of the following groups:

A. Infectious   (2 marks)

a. ....

b. ....

B. Non-infectious   (2 marks)

a. ....

b. ....

A lumbar puncture was performed. The CSF analysis showed:

RBC   35 cells/uL
WBC   120 cells/uL   (0–5)

predominantly lymphocytes

Protein   1.5 g/L   (0.15–0.45)

Glucose 2.7 mmol/L (Paired capillary blood glucose 8.3 mmol/L)

8.   **What empirical treatment would you prescribe if the CSF TB-PCR returns positive?**   (3 marks)

    ....

    ....

Question 10.4

A 27-year-old man, previously well, was seen for generalised body aches and pains for which he has been seeing various doctors over the last three years. One day, when attempting to climb a truck ladder, he felt his upper limb give way, and he fell.

1. **Give two possible reasons why he could possibly have felt his arms give way.** (2 marks)

    a. ....

    b. ....

After the fall he sustained a fracture; the X-ray is shown below:

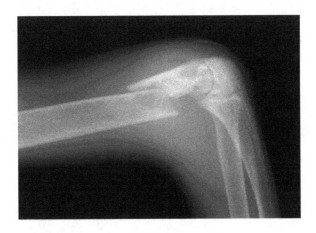

2.   Describe the important radiological finding(s). (2 marks)

....

....

3.   Based on the clinical presentation and radiological findings, which of the following are the LEAST likely considerations? Choose two. (2 marks)

    a. Cushing's syndrome
    b. Hyperparathyroidism
    c. Hypogonadism
    d. Multiple myeloma
    e. Osteogenesis imperfecta   (   ) & (   )

He gave a further history of polyuria and polydipsia over the past year.

4.   Which of the following are the LEAST likely conditions that explain this, given the aforesaid clinical context? Choose two. (2 marks)

    a. Diabetes mellitus
    b. Diuretic phase of acute renal failure
    c. Hyperparathyroidism
    d. Primary polydipsia
    e. Thyrotoxicosis   (   ) & (   )

On specific questioning, he had not taken any steroids or traditional medication. He has had a slight decrease in weight due to a poor appetite. Clinically he was normotensive, dehydrated and did not show any weight redistribution. He had normal secondary sexual characteristics.

5.   Which of the following are the MOST important investigations in view of these new findings? Choose two.

(2 marks)

   a. FSH, LH and testosterone levels
   b. Overnight dexamethasone suppression test and/or 24-hour urine free cortisol
   c. Protein electrophoresis
   d. Serum calcium, phosphate and albumin
   e. Urea, creatinine and electrolytes   (   ) & (   )

Of his laboratory investigations, his serum calcium level was noted to be 3.32 mmol/L (2.2–2.64).

6.   What is the added value of performing the following investigations?   (1 x 3 = 3 marks)

   A. Serum phosphate level

   ....

   B. Serum Vitamin D level

   ....

   C. Urinary calcium

   ....

This man was confirmed to have parathyroid adenoma based on a markedly elevated parathyroid hormone of 276 pmol/L (0.5–5.1). After fixation of the fracture, he underwent surgery to remove the adenoma. On the first post-operative day, he complained of severe cramps and pains in his muscles.

7.   What is the MOST likely explanation?   (1 mark)

   ....

8.   What is the MOST appropriate management?   (2 marks)

....

The X-ray below shows the man's left hand.

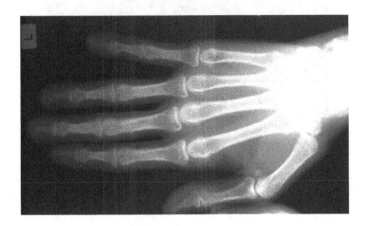

9.   Describe the radiological abnormality(s).   (2 marks)

....

....

10. In the light of all the investigation results so far, return to the elbow X-ray in Question 1 and study it carefully. What radiological abnormality do you notice that explains the fracture? What is its pathological significance?   (2 marks)

....

....

Clue: An identical feature is also seen in the jaw X-ray from the same patient:

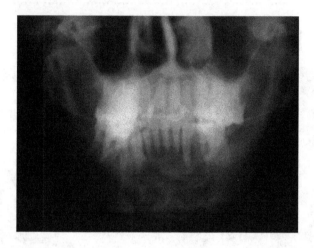

Question 10.5

A 20-year-old man who is currently undergoing national service presented to the emergency department with a complaint of bilateral leg swelling of one week's duration. It was associated with abdominal fullness and weight gain. He had no recent fever, chills or rashes. He denied any drug usage.

On physical examination, his pulse rate was 105/min and blood pressure 105/70 mmHg. Bilateral pitting oedema was present from his feet to mid-thighs. The abdomen was distended but no masses or tenderness were felt. His cardiorespiratory examination was normal.

1. **What specific history pertaining to his *urine* is helpful in the evaluation of this patient?** (2 marks)

    a. ....

    b. ....

2. **What is the relevance of taking a detailed sexual history?** (2 marks)

    ....

    ....

3.   What potential insights can you draw from a meticulous inspection of the jugular venous pressure?   (2 marks)

....

....

These are the results of the initial investigations.

Urine Dipstick:

Glucose	Negative
Ketones	Negative
Blood	Negative
Protein	3+
Bilirubin	Negative
Nitrite	Negative
Leucocytes	Negative

Renal panel:

Blood urea	4 mmol/L	(4.7–6.9)
Sodium	142 mmol/L	(135–145)
Potassium	3.9 mmol/L	(3.5–5)
Bicarbonate	20 mmol/L	(22–26)
Chloride	115 mmol/L	(95–105)
Serum creatinine	105 μmol/L	(70–100)
Calcium	2.45 mmol/L	(2.1–2.45)
Magnesium	0.85 mmol/L	(0.74–0.97)

Lipids profile:

Serum Total Cholesterol	11.94 mmol/L	(< 5.2)
Serum Cholesterol HDL	5.74 mmol/L	(1.0–1.5)
Serum Triglycerides	3.79 mmol/L	(1.7–2.2)
LDL (Calculated)	4.39 mmol/L	(2.6–3.3)

24-hour urine protein estimation:

    Urine Volume   2 litres

    Protein per Litre   4 grammes

    Total Protein   8 grammes

Ultrasonography of both kidneys:

    Normal size, bilateral

    Good cortical medullary differentiation

    Normal calyx and collecting systems

4.   What radiological investigation of the kidneys would you additionally order? Justify.   (2 marks)

....

....

A kidney biopsy showed epithelial cell injury and effacement of podocytes in almost the entire glomerulus.

5.   What is the complete diagnosis in this patient? (2 marks)

....

6A. What is the MOST specific intervention for this problem?   (2 marks)

....

6B. What adjunctive interventions may be considered at this stage?   (2 marks)

....

....

On the second evening of admission, the patient complained of breathlessness when the night nurse was taking his parameters. Oxygen saturation was 92% on room air.

7.   **Postulate two MOST likely causes of this acute development.**   (2 marks)

   a. ....

   b. ....

8.   **Give two investigations that you would order *immediately*.**
                                                                    (2 marks)

   a. ....

   b. ....

9.   **What are your nursing orders while awaiting your immediate investigations?**   (2 marks)

   ....

   ....

Solutions

Assessment Paper 1

1.1

1. Full neurological assessment (1). *If you write individual neuro-logical examination steps (e.g. tone testing, power of legs, pro-prioception sense, Romberg's sign, finger-nose test, etc.) as separate answers, these alone can take up ten (or more) answers — it wouldn't make much sense since you are only given four blanks! It would be more prudent to collapse them all so that you can examine other systems. Hence, if you mention two or more of each neurological step, you still will get a maximum of 1 mark. Ditto for "musculoskeletal examination".*
   Musculoskeletal examination (1)
   Gait assessment (1)
   Vision (1). *This includes acuity (day and night), peripheral fields, colour perception and glare tolerance.*
   Postural blood pressure (1)
   Cardiac auscultation for valvular disorders, e.g. mitral stenosis (0.5) — *less likely to directly cause falls but rather to evaluate the atrial fibrillation.*
   Anaemia (0.5)
   Signs of thyrotoxicosis (0.5) — *less likely to directly cause falls but rather to evaluate the atrial fibrillation*
   Timed up and go test (0) — *an example of a functional mobility test, which determines fall risk. It is not an assessment of aetiology.*
   (max. 4 marks)
2. Vitamin D level (1)
   Bone mineral density (1)

Cardiac workup, e.g. ECG, telemetry (0.5) — *arrhythmia as a cause for falls is less likely, as the atrial fibrillation in this scenario is chronic.*

Fasting glucose (0)

(max. 2 marks)

3. Hyperactive (0.5) delirium (0.5)

4A. Confusion Assessment Method (1)

4B. A and C (1)

5. Pain (1)

Medications (1) — *especially opiate analgesics*

Constipation (1) — *which could be contributed by opiate analgesics and being bedbound.*

Acute retention of urine (1) — *which could be contributed by all the above*

Dehydration (0.5)

Electrolyte abnormalities (0.5)

(max. 3 marks)

6. Immobility (1) leading to dependent oedema

Hypoalbuminaemia (1)

Deep vein thrombosis (1)

Fluid overload (0) — *would be accompanied by other signs, but her vital signs were stable.*

7. *Altered mental state in an elderly has many causes, but given the context of post-op hip replacement at one week, the following should be strongly considered:*

Nosocomial sepsis (1) — *such as urinary tract infection, pneumonia and wound infection*

Medications (1) — *such as analgesics and anti-psychotics*

Stroke (1) — *considering her age, cardiovascular risk factors (also AF!), post-op*

8. Swallowing assessment (1) — *post-stroke*

Rehabilitation potential (1) — *new motor stroke on the background of the recent femoral fracture post-op*

1.2

1. Rhythm abnormalities can signify a cardiac arrhythmia (1)
    Low volume pulse can signify hypovolaemia or aortic stenosis (1)
    Slow-rising (and slow-falling) pulse can signify aortic stenosis (1)
    Radiofemoral delay may suggest aortic atherosclerosis and indirectly carotid atherosclerosis (1)
    Bounding pulse may signify anaemia (1)
    Carotid bruit (0) — *carotid artery is not a "peripheral" pulse* (max. 3 marks)

2. Radiation of the cardiac murmur to neck (1)
    Palpable systolic thrill (1) — *e.g. severe aortic stenosis*
    Postural blood pressure (1)
    Clinical evidence of anaemia (conjunctiva, palmar creases and nailbeds) (1)
    Per rectal examination (1)
    Capillary blood glucose (1)
    Otoscopy (0.5) — *may be performed to rule out a peripheral cause such as chronic suppurative otitis media but this patient's symptoms improved with resting!*
    Dix–Hallpike test (0.5) — *should be performed with great caution in the elderly as they may have underlying cervical instability, vascular problems like vertebrobasilar insufficiency and carotid sinus syncope.*
    (max. 4 marks)

3A. Aortic valve calcification (1)

3B. Cardiomegaly OR left ventricular enlargement (1)
    Enlarged aortic knob (1)

4. Severe (1) aortic stenosis (1)

5. Heart failure (0.5)
    Pulmonary hypertension (0.5)
    Infective endocarditis (0.5)

Thromboembolic events (0.5)
Arrhythmias (0.5)
Angina (0.5)
(max. 2 marks)

6. B and C (1) — *in addition, diuretics should be judiciously used*

7. Aortic balloon dilatation
   Aortic valve replacement
   Aortic valve implantation — *as opposed to open-heart surgery for a valve replacement, this is performed via a transcatheter route.*
   (max. 2 marks)

8. Aspirin use
   Gastric ulcer
   Colorectal cancer
   Intestinal angiodysplasia — *a known association with aortic stenosis that gives rise to acquired von Willebrand deficiency = Heyde's syndrome*
   (max. 3 marks)

1.3

1. Scaly (0.5) erythematous (0.5) thickened (0.5) plaques (0.5) with ill-defined margins (0.5) and some crusting (0.5).
   (max. 2 marks)

2. C (1) — *apart from classical flexural predilection, nipples are an important site of involvement in atopic eczema.*

3. E (2)

4. C (1) — *hypertrichosis may, however, be present in some areas of excessive topical corticosteroid use.*

5. A (2) — *cream (or lotion) formulations are generally suitable for flexural dermatoses. Gels and solutions have alcoholic bases, which can cause irritation to acutely inflamed skin.*

Ointment formulation is generally suitable for lichenified or very thick lesions due to its occlusive property.

6. A and D (1 × 2 = 2 marks) — *one would tend to use a lower potency topical corticosteroid for lesions of shorter duration, on thinner regions of the body, and with acute inflammation.*

7. C (2)

8. D (2) — *hair dye dermatitis is usually a form of allergic contact dermatitis rather than irritant contact dermatitis, as in this case. By the time it presents, the morphology of allergic contact dermatitis would be characterised by scaliness, thickening and fissuring. For acute irritant dermatitis, erythema, oedema and oozing are typical features.*

9. C (2) — *all "wet" eczemas must be "dried" using astringent therapies like potassium permanganate soaks (or compresses). This amazing therapy functions as an astringent, antiseptic, cleanser and deodorant.*

10. B (2) — *the presence of monomorphic circular erosions (because all the vesicles have "broken down" from scratching) on a background of poorly controlled atopic eczema is highly suggestive.*

11. C (1)

12. D (1) — *azathioprine and methotrexate are not recommended for women planning a pregnancy. Hypertension is a relative contraindication for ciclosporin. Long-term systemic steroid is best avoided unless one has run out of options.*

1.4

1. Diabetic ketocidosis (1) as evidenced by raised glucose and serum ketones and a metabolic acidosis (1)
    This is not a hyperosmolar hyperglycaemic state (HHS) (1), as one would expect the glucose, serum sodium and osmolality to

be higher (1). *Patients with HHS are likely to be obtunded, but this patient's GCS is 15.*

(max. 3 marks)

2. The serum bicarbonate is not as low as expected in diabetic ketoacidosis (DKA) (1) because of her severe frequent vomiting, which led to a loss of hydrogen ions in gastric content (1).

3. A, E and F ($1 \times 3 = 3$ marks)

4. Hourly (1) to allow for titration for IV insulin dose (1) and monitoring of response to treatment (1)

    (max 2 marks)

5A. *Despite a normal potassium level*, IV potassium (1) should be started concurrently with the IV insulin because insulin will cause the potassium to enter the cells (1), *potentially causing life-threatening arrhythmias!*

    Oral potassium (0)

5B. 4–6 hourly (1)

6. Sudden discontinuation of IV insulin can cause a rebound of DKA (1) as IV insulin is very short-acting (1).

7. Basal bolus (1) allows flexibility (1) *whereas, with premixed insulin, meal times and frequency have to be very regular.*

8A. Tremors (0.5)

    Sweating (0.5)

    Palpitations (0.5)

    Blurring of vision (0.5)

    Confusion (0.5)

    Dizziness (0.5)

    (max. 2 marks)

8B. Take 15 g of fast-acting carbohydrate (1) *and recheck sugar level in 15 minutes. Examples of fast-acting carbohydrates are glucose tablets, glucose or non-diet soft drinks, orange juice, and sweets.*

1.5

1. B (1) — *any primary source of sepsis? As we shall see later (as the underlying diagnosis becomes apparent), pulmonary haemorrhage and acute respiratory distress syndrome are some important things to look for too (a retrospective consideration).*

2. *Given the information provided so far, the three most important considerations at this stage are*: sepsis (1), hyponatraemia (1) and subtherapeutic carbamazepine levels due to poor compliance or vomiting (1).
    Other possible considerations are: hypoglycaemia (0.5), obstructive sleep apnoea (0.5) and meningitis (0.5)
    (max. 3 marks)

3. E (1) — *all the options are possible causes of "troponin leak", but option E is the most reasonable in this setting. Sepsis and rhabdomyolysis are also important considerations.*

4. A (2) — *this patient is at significant risk of acute kidney injury from septic shock and rhabdomyolysis. You can reduce the risk by improving mean arterial pressure to above 90 mmHg with aggressive hydration (and inotropic support if required). Early and aggressive fluid resuscitation is the most important preventive strategy for anyone with an elevated creatine kinase (CK) of more than 5,000 units/L. The rate of fluid administration is adjusted to achieve the desired diuresis of 200–300 ml/hr. Normal saline can be used for volume replacement. Limited data suggests the benefit of urinary alkalinisation with isotonic bicarbonate, but beware of alkalosis and discontinue if arterial pH increases to 7.5, serum bicarbonate exceeds 30 mmol/L or if symptomatic hypocalcaemia develops.*

5A. D (1) — *urine myoglobin is commonly done to support the diagnosis of rhabdomyolysis but note that the test is insensitive and expensive. In the relevant clinical setting, positive haem on a Dipstick combined with the absence of red blood cells (RBCs) in a Urine Full Examination Microscopic Examination*

(UFEME) is sufficient evidence to make the diagnosis of rhabdomyolysis.

5B. B (1) — *muscle enzymes like lactate dehydrogenase (LDH), aspartate aminotransferase (AST), alanine aminotransferase (ALT) and aldolase will be elevated but note that testing all these is not necessary for diagnosis. It is important to remember that elevation of these enzymes can be secondary to muscle damage in the setting of rhabdomyolysis so that initiation of unnecessary tests for liver and cardiac pathologies can be avoided. You can get false negative plasma myoglobin levels because it has a short half-life and thus is cleared from plasma within a few hours.*

6. C (1) — *transient hypocalcaemia is often seen in rhabdomyolysis due to calcium deposition in injured tissues. As there is a risk of late occurrence of hypercalcaemia and the risk of calcium phosphate precipitation, treatment of hypocalcaemia should be avoided unless the patient is symptomatic.*

7. Continuous renal replacement therapy (CRRT) (1). *Renal replacement therapy is indicated for the management of hyperkalaemia, fluid overload, metabolic acidosis and uraemia in a patient with established acute kidney injury. In this clinical setting,* **as the patient is haemodynamically unstable, and on inotropic support,** *CRRT is the ideal choice. Even though there is a theoretical advantage of CRRT over conventional haemodialysis in rhabdomyolysis and acute kidney injury, there is insufficient clinical evidence to support its use over conventional haemodialysis in patients who are haemodynamically stable.*

8. *Given the information provided so far, the three most important considerations at this stage are:* prolonged post-ictal state (1), cerebrovascular accident (1) and meningoencephalitis (1). *Other possible considerations are:* non-convulsive seizures (1) and undiagnosed drug poisoning (1)
Inappropriate possibilities are: hepatic encephalopathy (0), renal failure (0) and hyperphosphataemia (0)
(max. 3 marks)

Although meningitis and encephalitis are the most likely based on fever, raised inflammatory marks and haemodynamic instability, this patient also has significant cardiovascular risk factors — she can still have a cerebrovascular accident despite a normal CT scan of her brain! An MRI should be ordered.

9A. Traumatic tap (1) — *not subarachnoid haemorrhage as a CT brain scan showed no bleed*

Not xanthochromic (1) — *as would be seen in subarachnoid haemorrhage*

Meningitis (1) — *increased opening pressure, high protein*

Less likely bacterial OR more likely viral/aseptic (1) — *fluid is clear, white blood cells not particularly high, gram stain negative, and meningitis multiplex-PCR negative (for Streptococcus pneumoniae, Streptococcus agalactiae, Neisseria meningitides and Haemophilus influenzae)*

(max. 3 marks)

9B. CSF glucose level (1). This is typically low in bacterial meningitis and normal in most viral meningitis.

10. *Leptospira sp* (1). *It caused acute meningoencephalitis with rhabdomyolysis and acute kidney injury in this patient. Conjunctival suffusion, characterised by conjunctival redness and subconjunctival haemorrhage are important signs of leptospirosis, which were present in this case. The presence of hepatitis with jaundice and thrombocytopenia are the other features that should raise suspicion. Rhabdomyolysis is well known to occur in leptospirosis, but this is not the only mechanism of renal failure. Renal failure due to leptospirosis is often nonoliguric, and it can be associated with hypokalaemia, which suggests significant tubulointerstitial pathology.*

11. Pulmonary haemorrhage (1)

Acute respiratory distress syndrome (1)

Pulmonary embolism (0)

(max. 1 mark)

Assessment Paper 2

2.1

1A. Pre-eclampsia/HELLP (Haemolysis, Elevated Liver enzyme levels, and Low Platelet levels) syndrome. (1)

1B. Oedema (1)

> **PLUS**
>
> Any sign(s) of pulmonary congestion (1): e.g. tachypnea, basal crepitations
>
> Any sign(s) of haemolysis (1): e.g. jaundice, anaemia
>
> Any sign(s) of dehydration from excessive vomiting (1): e.g. dry mucous membranes
>
> Papilloedema (0) — *highly unlikely as she has no ocular complaint*
>
> (max. 2 marks)

1C. A, D, G and H ($0.5 \times 4 = 2$ marks)

2. Chronic gastrointestinal tract blood loss (1)

Anaemia in pregnancy (1)

Inadequate iron intake (1)

Haemolysis (0) *is not evident from the history*

3. C (2)

4A. Iron deficiency (2) *as indicated by the hypochromic microcytic anaemia with high red cell distribution width, low ferritin and transferrin saturation.*

4B. A (2). *Although high-dose oral iron replacement would be a first line option, intravenous iron may be indicated if oral replacement is inadequate or intolerable.*

5.

A: Differential Diagnosis (max. 2 marks)	B: Investigation/ Intervention for Evaluation (max. 2 marks)
Pseudothrombocytopaenia (1) — *a laboratory artefact due to platelet clumping induced by EDTA*	Repeat platelet count using a heparin or sodium citrate collection tube (1)
Cirrhosis (1) *resulting in splenic sequestration*	Ultrasound abdomen (1) *to evaluate for possible cirrhosis/splenomegaly*
Immune-mediated thrombocytopenia (1) *possibly secondary to Helicobactor pylori infection*	Treat *Helicobactor pylori* and repeat platelet count after *Helicobactor pylori* eradication (1)

2.2

1A. Supraventricular tachycardia (1)
     Narrow complex tachycardia (0.5)
     (max. 1 mark)
1B. IV adenosine (1) *is the drug of choice because while it is as effective as verapamil, it is far less toxic (due to extremely short half-life).*
         PLUS
         IV verapamil (1)
         IV procainamide (1)
         IV beta-blocker (propranolol, metoprolol) (1)
         IV amiodarone (1)
         (max. 1 mark)

2. For a *differential diagnosis, consider the context of a returned traveller with fever, headache and pancytopenia.*

	Differential Diagnosis	Diagnostic Investigation (max. 1 mark for each box)
A	Malaria	Malarial blood film
B	Dengue fever	Dengue antigen (EIA), blood dengue virus PCR/viral load
C	Chikungunya	Chikungunya IgM
D	Zika virus infection	Blood Zika virus PCR or urine Zika virus PCR
E	Leptospirosis	Leptospira IgM or urine Leptospira PCR
F	Rickettsial infection	Rickettsial serology
G	Sepsis due to bacteraemia	Blood culture
H	Meningitis	Lumbar puncture

(max. 4 marks)

3. *Plasmodium vivax* (1) malaria (1)

4A. B (2) — *any of these combinations would be appropriate:*
Artemether + lumefantrine (ACT) (3 days)
Artesunate + amodiaquine (ACT) (3 days)
Artesunate + mefloquine (ACT) (3 days)
Atovaquone-proguanil (malarone) (3 days)
Quinine + doxycycline or clindamycin (7 days)
Artesunate + foxycycline or clindamycin (7 days)
Note: Plasmodium vivax has shown chloroquine resistance in Papua New Guinea and Indonesia.

4B. Primaquine (1) to eradicate the dormant hypnozoites (liver stages of *P vivax*) (1).

5. Hepatitis A vaccination (1)
    Hepatitis B vaccination (1)
    Malaria prophylaxis (1)
    Typhoid vaccination (1)
    Rabies vaccination (1)
    Japanese encephalitis vaccination (1)
    (max. 3 marks)

2.3

1. Scaly (0.5) crusted (0.5) erythematous (0.5) papules (0.5) and
    plaques (0.5) with fissuring (0.5)
    (max. 2 marks)
2. Allergic contact dermatitis (1)
    Irritant contact dermatitis (0)
3. Contact with cement (1)
    Contact with traditional Chinese medication (1)
    Contact with asbestos (0) — *asbestos-induced contact dermatitis
    is extremely rare, and if it happens, is due to airborne asbestos
    particles inducing a reaction on the exterior surfaces of skin that
    likely encounter the particles. Such areas typically include the
    cheeks and neck.*
4. A (2) — *do not confuse patch testing with prick testing — the
    latter is a test for immediate allergic reactions.*
5. C (1)
6A. Calcified linear shadows over both diaphragms (1)
    "Holly leaf" shaped opacity over right middle-lower zones (1).
    *Pleural plaques are a common manifestation of asbestos expo-
    sure. They can be calcified or non-calcified, and are commonly
    found on the posterolateral aspect of the chest wall and over
    diaphragmatic domes. The holly leaf appearance results from
    the plaques having thickened rolled margins.*

6B. Diffuse pleural opacities (1) — *which may signify pleural thickening or mesothelioma*
Pleural effusion (1)
Parenchymal opacity (1) — *which may signify bronchogenic carcinoma*
Pulmonary fibrosis (1)
(max. 2 marks)
Note: The question specifically asks for radiological findings, so you should not offer clinical or histological diagnoses.

7. Occupational history (1) — *although construction work puts him at high risk of developing asbestosis, it is important to check if he has also worked in other high-risk industries, e.g. plumbing, ship-building and electrical works.*
History of tuberculosis (1) — *especially that of pleural TB*
History of trauma with haemothorax (1)
History of pleural interventions, e.g. talc pleurodesis (1)
(max. 3 marks)

8. Asbestos-related pleural plaques (1)
Pleural plaques (1) typically affect the lower aspects (1) of lungs found in a patient who developed symptoms 20 years (1) after occupational exposure.
(max. 3 marks)

9. B and C ($1 \times 2 = 2$ marks) — *the earliest pulmonary function abnormality is a decreased diffusion capacity*

2.4

1A. ***Enlarged painful kidney and fever*:**
Right pyelonephritis (0.5) with hydronephrosis/pyonephrosis/perinephric abscess/renal carbuncle (0.5)
Emphysematous pyelonephritis (1)
Polycystic kidney disease (0.5) with an infected kidney cyst (0.5)
(max. 2 marks)

1B. **Acutely enlarged painful kidney without fever:**

Acute renal vein thrombosis (2) *usually occurs in hypercoagulable states, e.g. nephrotic syndrome, but it more frequently occurs on the left side, as the vein is longer than the right.*

Haemorrhage (1) in renal angiomylolipoma (1), *but this occurs more frequently in middle-aged females with tuberose sclerosis.*

Spontaneous perinephric haemorrhage (2) *is most commonly due to an underlying renal neoplasm.*

Renal cell carcinoma (1) *more likely to present with enlarged testicle (testicular metastasis or varicocoele due to renal vein thrombosis) than an enlarged kidney; a fever may uncommonly be a paraneoplastic phenomenon.*

Infiltrative conditions, e.g. amyloidosis (0) *would not have an acute presentation.*

(max. 2 marks)

2. **Any male urinary tract infection (UTI) is complicated let alone an upper tract infection! Further evaluation (of predisposing factors, previous workup and previous management) is always needed:**

History of obstructive urinary tract symptoms (0.5)

History of sexually transmitted infections (0) *is correct as urethral stenosis is a possible sequala of Gonorrhea and Chlamydia infections, but it would present as obstructive urinary tract symptoms, so this answer is subsumed under it.*

Presence of lower UTI symptoms (0.5)

History of kidney stones (0.5)

History of recent instrumentation (0.5)

Family history of polycystic kidney disease (0.5)

Family history of urinary tract abnormalities (0) *is also correct, but this would more likely have presented at a younger age.*

Degree of control of diabetes (0.5)

Investigations performed when he developed UTI prior to admission (0.5)

Treatment received when he developed UTI prior to admission (0.5)

(max. 3 marks)

3. Acute kidney injury in the background of chronic kidney disease OR acute-on-chronic kidney disease (1)

High anion-gap (0.5) metabolic acidosis (0.5)

4. Multiple (0.5) renal cysts (0.5) of varying sizes (0.5) in both (0.5) kidneys, some with internal echoes and wall calcification (0.5).

(max. 2 marks)

5. Adequate hydration (1) — *intravenously if the patient is unable to tolerate orally*

Antibiotic with superior penetration into kidney cysts (1) — *such as fluoroquinolones*

Monitoring and control of blood glucose (1)

Symptomatic management (0.5) — *e.g. antipyrexial medication and pain medication are both important but of lower priority than the above three.*

Sodium replacement (0)

(max. 3 marks)

6. **Disease progression** (1) (of autosomal dominant polycystic kidney disease): inevitable — once he has been treated for the acute infection, the kidney function may achieve a *new baseline*.

Disease progression **can be delayed** (1): by control of risk factors such as *hypertension*

Disease has **extra-renal manifestations** (1): *cerebral aneurysm, liver cyst and cardiac valvular lesions* that need evaluation if there are significant signs and symptoms.

Disease heritability (1): **Screening** for family members, in particular, his *children*, is strongly encouraged.

7. Ruptured berry aneurysm with subarachnoid haemorrhage (1)
    Renal artery stenosis secondary to compression from renal
    cysts (1)
    Intracerebral haemorrhage from a ruptured Charcot Bouchard
    aneurysm due to these risk factors: age, hypertension, chronic
    kidney disease, etc (1).
    (max. 2 marks)

2.5

1A. F and G (1 × 2 = 2 marks) — *this patient has persistent hyper-*
    tension, hypokalaemia, kaliuresis and metabolic alkalosis.
    Bartter and Liddle syndromes would have manifested by ado-
    lescents; in any case, patients with Bartter syndrome are usu-
    ally normotensive (due to salt-wasting). Concomitant
    hypochloraemia would be expected with diuretic use.
1B. Aldosterone: Renin ratio (1) *would distinguish between pri-*
    mary and secondary aldosteronism. High aldosterone and low
    renin levels are suggestive of primary aldosteronism (0.5); high
    aldosterone and high renin levels are suggestive of renal artery
    stenosis (0.5).
    Duplex ultrasound of renal arteries (0) — *is only good to*
    screen for renal artery stenosis. A negative ultrasound does
    not automatically rule in primary aldosteronism.
2A. Obstructive sleep apnoea (1) due to obesity (1)
2B. Polysomnography OR overnight sleep study (1)
    Epworth sleepiness scale and STOP-BANG (0) *are question-*
    naires not investigations
3A. D (2) — *"total" refers to a combination of a higher cerebral*
    dysfunction (i.e., dysphasia, dyscalculia, visuospatial disor-
    der), homonymous visual field defect, and motor and/or sen-
    sory deficit of at least two areas of the face, arm and leg;
    "partial" refers to two of these three components.

3B. Left (1) middle cerebral artery (1) ± anterior cerebral artery (0.5) (max. 2 marks)
4. A (2) — *as the timing of onset of the stroke is unknown, he is not eligible for thombolytic therapy.*
5. MRI/MRA brain (1)
    PLUS
    Doppler ultrasound carotid arteries (1)
    24-hour Holter (1)
    Transthoracic echocardiography (1)
    Any young stroke workup (0)
    (max. 2 marks)
6. Systolic blood pressure (BP) >220 mmHg (1) OR Diastolic BP >120 mmHg (1)
7. Urinary catheterisation (1). Check and treat its cause (1), e.g. faecal loading due to constipation. *Only after all the reversible causes have been managed should one consider pharmacological treatment.*

Assessment Paper 3

3.1

1. Autonomic neuropathy (1) *due to Parkinson's disease and diabetes*
    Medications (1) — *anti-hypertensives, medication for benign prostatic hypertrophy (BPH)*
    Dehydration (1) *from poor oral intake*
2. Romberg's test (1) *can identify vestibular dysfunction, provided his vision and proprioception are intact.*
    Cerebellar examination (1)
    Cranial nerve examination (1) *to look for brainstem vascular lesion or progressive supranuclear palsy*

Fluid status assessment (1)

Cardiovascular assessment (0.5) — *pulses, bruits, murmurs*

Capillary blood glucose (0) *is a biochemical assessment, not a "clinical" assessment.*

Hearing assessment (0) — *if impaired may suggest Meniere disease but that is a gradual progressive disorder that happens over time, not just two weeks.*

Otoscopy (0) *can identify chronic suppurative otitis media but that is associated with vertigo lasting more than six weeks; acute otitie media causes otalgia, not giddiness.*

(max. 3 marks)

3.   Intravenous hydration (1)

Stop anti-hypertensives (0.5) including tamsulosin (0.5)

Stop oral hypoglycaemic agents (1) — *in view of low blood sugar, low HbA1c and acute kidney impairment*

Any measure to reduce serum potassium (0)

4.   Fasting blood glucose (1)

8 am Cortisol (0) — *to assess for adrenal insufficiency in view of low sodium level may appear to be a good thought but the clinical picture is not that of hypoadrenalism, particularly in the context of dehydration; a person with cortisol deficiency would not just have two weeks' history of giddiness.*

Fasting lipids (0) *is a test that should be performed in a primary care setting*

5.   Dopamine agonist (1)

Monoamine-oxidase B inhibitor (1)

Catechol-O-methyltransferase inhibitor (1)

Amantadine (0.5) *is a specific tricyclic amine antiviral that is probably more useful as an adjunct therapy to dopamine agonist in Parkinson disease, although it has also been touted as a dopamine agonist-sparing agent in early diseases.*

(max. 3 marks)

6A. *The patient was most likely started on Madopar (a combination of levodopa and benserazide). Benserazide inhibits the peripheral decarboxylation of levodopa. Postural hypotension is a common adverse reaction.*

Decrease Madopar to its lowest effective dose (1)

Change to another class of drugs (1)

6B. Compression stockings (1)

Increase water intake (1)

Physical counter-manoeuvres, e.g. standing up slowly, leg crossing, buttock clenching (1)

Abdominal binders (1)

Sleeping with head of bed raised 30–45 degrees (1)

Increase salt intake (0) — *note the background of hypertension!*

(max. 2 marks)

7. E (2) — *look closely at the scaly annular edge traversing down from the right face over to the right trapezius*

8. Telangiectasias (1)

Atrophy (0) — *not visible from these photographs*

3.2

1. Gout (1) — *metatarsophalangeal joint monoarthritis is classic for gout, especially if episodes have been recurrent.*

   PLUS

   Septic arthritis (1) — *this is the most important differential to rule out acutely*

   Gonococcal arthritis (1) — *important cause of acute monoarthritis, though less frequently in smaller joints.*

   Rheumatoid arthritis (0.5) — *may be an unusual first presentation*

   Psoriatic arthritis (0.5) — *may be an unusual first presentation*

Pseudogout (0.5) — *less likely to present at the first metatarsophalangeal joint, more likely at large joints, e.g., knee.*

Haemarthrosis (0) — without antecedent trauma is extremely uncommon

(max. 2 marks)

2. Arthrocentesis with synovial fluid analysis (1)

Serum uric acid level (1): *if the level is high, it is helpful; low or normal levels do not exclude gout, so this should be rechecked at least two weeks after the gouty attack has resolved.*

X-ray left foot (1) *to look for periarticular erosions, but one is more likely to find soft tissue swelling in this case of the first episode of gouty attack.*

(max. 2 marks)

3. Polycythaemia vera (2)

4. Systemic hypoxia, e.g. chronic smoking, obstructive sleep apnoea, *prolonged exposure to high altitudes, chronic lung disease, less likely cyanotic heart disease at this age.*

Paraneoplastic production of erythropoietin, e.g. renal cell carcinoma, hepatocellular carcinoma, cerebellar hemangioblastoma, benign lesions such as leiomyoma and renal cysts.

(max. 4 marks)

5A. Erythromelalgia (1)

Raynaud phenomenon (0) *will present with a sudden whitening of the skin due to arterial spasms in response to cold exposure followed by reactive hyperaemia*

5B. This is due to vaso-occlusion of the small blood vessels in the extremities (1), followed by intense hyperaemia (0.5) and burning pain. This can happen in myeloproliferative disorders, which are prothrombotic conditions (1).

6. Pancytosis OR panmyelosis (1)

7. Antiplatelet drug, e.g. aspirin (1)

Cytoreductive therapy, e.g. hydroxyurea (1)

Colchicine (1) *for acute gouty attack*

Nonsteroidal anti-inflammatory drug (NSAID) (1) *for acute gouty attack*
Allopurinol (0)
(max. 2 marks)

8. Whitish deposits over several joints (1)
Bulbous swelling over the proximal metacarpophalangeal joint of left middle finger (1)

9. Check renal function, as the dose may need to be titrated (1)
   PLUS
   Counsel patient to watch for rashes and to seek medical attention immediately if rashes appear (1)
   PLUS
   Send blood for genotyping of HLA-B*5801 (1) — *to determine risk for the development of Stevens Johnson syndrome with allopurinol; note that this may not be widely available*
   Concurrent low-dose colchicine (1) to prevent flare during initiation of allopurinol
   Consider drug interactions with allopurinol (1)
   (max. 1 mark)

3.3

1. Apex beat (1)
   Radioradial OR radiofemoral delay OR pulse asynchrony (1)
   Differential blood pressure of the arm and leg (1)
   Peripheral pulses examination (1)
   Blood pressure of the leg (0.5)
   Abdominal bruit (or renal bruit) OR arterial bruit (1)
   (max. 2 marks)

2. Prognathism (1)
   Malocclusion (1)
   Thickened lips (1)
   Prominent nasolabial folds (1)

Prominent supraorbital ridge (1)

Coarse facial features (max. 1 mark) — viz. broad nose (0.5), interdental separation OR splaying of teeth (0.5).

Acne scars (0.5) — *suggestive of a history of severe acne, which may indicate excessive androgenic influence; however, acne on its own is a very common skin disorder in the population.*

Frontal hairline recession (0.5): *suggestive of excessive androgenic influence; however, androgenetic alopecia on its own is a very common phenomenon in the population.*

(max. 2 marks)

PLUS

Large hands with broad fingers OR widening of fingers (1)

3. Frontal bossing (1)

Maxillary (or cheekbone) widening or prominence (1)

Squaring of jaw (1)

Nasolabial fold prominence (1)

Thickening of lower lips (1)

(max. 1 mark)

4A. Confrontational visual field testing (1): *to look for bitemporal hemianopia, which would likely indicate compression of the optic chiasm from a pituitary adenoma.*

Testing of power in the upper and lower limbs (0.5) *may reveal proximal myopathy. While this is a recognised feature of acromegaly, it is a non-specific feature.*

Testing for sensory loss in the median nerve distribution, wasting of the LOAF (lateral two lumbricals, opponent pollicis, abductor pollicis brevis, flexor pollicis brevis) muscles, and Hoffman-Tinel and Phalen signs (0.5) *are consistent with carpal tunnel syndrome. Bilateral carpal tunnel syndrome is a well-recognised feature of acromegaly, but again, these are non-specific signs and would not indicate the presence of an underlying pituitary adenoma.*

(max. 1 mark)

4B. Goitre (1)
Acanthosis nigricans (1)
Skin tags (1)
(max. 2 marks)

5. It is inappropriate as growth hormone (GH) secretion is pulsatile (1). *Random sampling results in both false-positive and false-negative results. Patients can have the active disease (acromegaly) even though GH levels fall within the normal range. If the basal growth hormone level is extremely high, e.g. 100 mIU/L, then it is strongly suggestive of acromegaly.*

6. While GH excess induces insulin resistance and as many as 50% of patients may have a form of dysglycaemia on an oral glucose tolerance test, there was **no evidence of diabetes mellitus or impaired fasting glucose or impaired glucose tolerance.** (1)
The oral glucose tolerance test showed the **failure of adequate suppression of GH in response to a glucose load**. (1) The nadir in the level of GH was elevated at 11 mIU/L in this patient, which confirms acromegaly.
The GH acts by inducing the synthesis of IGF-1 predominantly by the liver. Therefore, IGF-1 is representative of average daily GH secretion, and levels remain stable throughout the day. In this patient, the **elevated IGF-1 reflects the hypersecretion of GH** (1), which is consistent with acromegaly.

7. Serum parathyroid hormone level (1). *Primary hyperparathyroidism causing hypercalcaemia has high penetrance and is almost invariably the first manifestation of MEN 1 and therefore is a useful and easy biochemical screening investigation. This consideration is important, particularly in a patient presenting at this age (35 years old).*

8. C (2) — *remember the mnemonic: **MEN 1 = 3 Ps (Pituitary, Parathyroid, Pancreas)**! MEN 2 is associated with medullary thyroid cancer, parathyroid adenoma and pheochromocytoma, but not pituitary adenoma. The Von Hippel–Lindau syndrome is*

an inherited disease characterised by retinal and cranial haemanioblastomas and pheochromocytoma, but not acromegaly or hypercalcaemia from primary hyperparathyroidism.

9. (2)

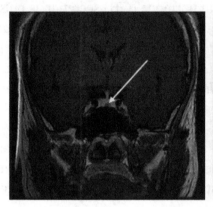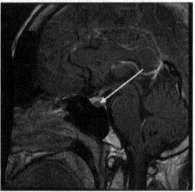

10. Somatostatin analogue (1), *e.g. octreotide, lanreotide, pasireotide*
    Dopamine agonist (1), *e.g. cabergoline*
    GH receptor antagonist (1), *e.g. pegvisomant*
    Radiotherapy (1)
    (max. 2 marks)
11. Colonoscopy (1)
    Stool occult blood (0.5)
    Full blood count (0.5)
    (max. 1 mark)
    Patients with acromegaly are at increased risk for malignancies, especially colorectal cancer. Most guidelines recommend a colonoscopy at the time of diagnosis of acromegaly. Stool occult blood and full blood count (FBC) are inferior to colonoscopy for the screening of colorectal cancer. The interval for a follow-up colonoscopy has not been firmly established. You may also wish to note that cabergoline can cause constipation as a side effect.

3.4

1. Hepatic encephalopathy (1)
   Sepsis (1)
   Medications causing confusion/constipation (1), e.g. benzodiazepines, anticholinergics and opiates
   Hypoxia (1)
   Undiagnosed brain metastases (1)
   Hypercalcaemia or hyponatraemia (0) *are electrolyte disturbances, which are specifically to be excluded in question*
   Ureamia (0) *is already implied to be looked for in the question*
   (max. 3 marks)

2A. Typical antipsychotics such as haloperidol (1)
   Atypical antipsychotics such as risperidone and quetiapine (1)
   Be cognizant of drug interactions, e.g. benzodiazepines such as lorazepam should NOT be used as a single agent as it may cause paradoxical agitation, but it can be used in combination with an antipsychotic for more rapid sedation of the agitated delirious patient.
   (max. 1 mark)

2B. Frequent re-orientation (1)
   Presence of family members or familiar items from home (1)
   (max. 1 mark)

3. Establish goals of care, discuss extent of care and resuscitation status with the family (1)
   Discontinue inappropriate investigations, interventions and medications (1), *e.g. blood tests, radiological scans and frequent parameter checking.*
   Prescribe medications to control symptoms (1)
   Oral, skin, bladder and bowel care (1)
   (max. 3 marks)

4.   D (2) — *the medical team is not obligated to provide medically futile treatment*

5.   D (2) — *the ACP document allows the patient to express his preferences, which can be taken into account when making medical decisions. However, it is not legally binding. The medical team is still not obligated to provide medically futile treatment.*

6.   Potential benefits of hydration and/or nutrition (1), *e.g. preventing or treating symptoms that may be caused by dehydration such as lethargy or delirium.*

Potential harms of hydration and/or nutrition (1), *e.g. increasing peripheral and pulmonary oedema, risk of infection or aspiration.*

Potential burdens of hydration and/or nutrition (1), *e.g. discomfort of intravenous access of the feeding tube.*

Meaning of hydration and nutrition to patient and/or family (1): *is it perceived as a basic provision of food and water, a source of support and a symbol of caring?*

(max. 2 marks)

7A. Anti-cholinergic medications (1), *e.g. subcutaneous/intravenous hyoscine butylbromide 20 mg stat + 20 mg TDS*

7B. Reposition the patient (1), *e.g. propped up or in a lateral position*

Reduce or stop subcutaneous/intravenous fluids (or NG feeds if being given) (1)

Gentle suctioning only if patient is able to tolerate without too much discomfort (1)

The family should be reassured that as distressing as it may appear, most patients are not bothered by the respiratory tract secretions.

(max. 1 mark)

8.   B (2) — *administer a stat dose of subcutaneous haloperidol for pharmacological management of terminal restlessness. Typical*

starting doses are subcutaneous haloperidol (0.5–1 mg BD/
TDS) and 0.5–1 mg up to every 4–6 hours as needed.
9. Cognitive changes, e.g. delirium (1)
   Low blood pressure that is not related to hypovolaemia (1)
   Loss of ability to close one's eyes (1)
   Hallucinations involving previously deceased relatives (1)
   Respiratory tract secretions (1)
   Altered respiratory pattern (1)
   Mottling and cooling of skin, starting in the peripheries (1)
   Profound progressive weakness (1)
   Loss of interest and/or ability to drink/eat (1)
   (max. 2 marks)

3.5

1. Respiratory compensation for lactic acidosis due to tissue
   hypoperfusion (1)
   Stimulation of medullary respiratory centre by bacterial endo-
   toxins and/or other inflammatory mediators (1)
   Pulmonary embolism or any other chest disorder (0)
2. *This is really a question on the principles of management in*
   septic shock, so specific details are not needed at this stage:
   Check airway, breathing and circulation (1)
   Aggressive fluid/haemodynamic resuscitation (1)
   Close monitoring of parameters (1)
   Evaluation of organ function (1)
   Blood cultures and early and adequate antibiotics (1)
   Source control (0.5)
   (max. 5 marks)
3A. Insert two (0.5) large-bore (0.5) intravenous cannulae to infuse 30
    ml/kg (1–2L) (0.5) crystalloid fluid (e.g. 0.9% sodium chloride,
    Hartman's solution) (0.5) rapidly over 30–60 minutes (0.5).
    (max. 2 marks)

3B. Inotropic support (0.5) with intravenous noradrenaline (0.5) via a central line (0.5) at 5–20 mcg/min (0.5) in the intensive care unit (0.5).

Dopamine (0) *is not a first-line inotropic agent as it may cause tachyarrhythmias*

(max. 2 marks)

4. Vaccination history of tetanus (1) *because tetanus immuno-globulin is needed if there are less than three previous immunisations.*

History of liver disease (1) *because it is a major risk factor for Vibrio vulnificus infection*

Presence of iron overload states (1), *e.g. thalassaemia major requiring repeated blood transfusions, and haemachromatosis because it is also a major risk factor for Vibrio vulnificus infection*

History of peripheral vascular disease (1) *as it may affect the surgical decision of debridement versus amputation.*

History of splenectomy (1) *would suggest the infective agent to be an encapsulated organism.*

(max. 2 marks)

5A. A combination of one gram-positive cover, one gram-negative (must encompass anti-*Pseudomonas* activity in view of the water exposure history) cover and one anaerobic cover is the treatment of choice in necrotising fasciitis. So ideally, you would want to give vancomycin (0.5) + ceftazidime OR fluoroquinolone (e.g. ciprofloxacin) (0.5) + metronidazole OR clindamycin (0.5). As *Vibrio vulnificus is strongly suspected here — note the additional risk factors of poorly controlled diabetes and* **chronic alcoholism** *— you should add* oral doxycycline (0.5), *as the combination of ceftazidime/doxycycline is ideal for this pathogen. If you had earlier written a fluoquinolone or a carbapenem such as imipenem or meropenem (but*

NOT ertapenem as it does not cover Pseudomonas well) in place of ceftazidime, then doxycycline is also not necessary. Although this patient has a possible history of penicillin allergy, one's consideration for a third-generation cephalosporin must give strong weightage to the life-threatening nature of this infection and the negligible risk of cross-reaction with penicillin.

Any penicillin (0) *is contraindicated from the history of possible penicillin allergy*

IVIG (0) *is controversial*

(max. 2 marks)

5B. Urgent surgical debridement (2) *is life-saving!*

6. What exactly were the symptoms (and severity)? (1)

Has he ever developed a similar rash in the absence of penicillin? (1)

How long ago did the reaction occur? (1) *This question is important because the subsequent risk of immediate hypersensitivity reactions decreases with time (immunological waning).*

Had penicillin been used before the reported adverse drug reaction? (1)

Did the reaction occur within minutes, hours or days of consuming penicillin? (1)

Were other medications used concurrently at the time of the reaction? (1)

Did he tolerate any other similar medication taken since then, such as amoxicillin, amoxicillin-clavulanate and first-generation cephalosporin? (1)

Has the "allergy" been formally assessed by a specialist (or investigated with skin prick test, challenge, etc.)? (1)

(max. 3 marks)

Assessment Paper 4

4.1

1. Osteoarthritis of knees/hips/spine (1)
   Daytime somnolence (1) *due to obstructive sleep apnoea*
   Postural instability (1) *due to more rapid sway, greater tendency to slip sideways and other mechanical factors*
   Peripheral neuropathy due to diabetes (1)
   (max. 2 marks)
2A. Purplish striae (1)
   Easy bruising (1)
   Atrophic skin (1) — *these three features found in Cushing's syndrome. In addition, dry thin wrinkled skin (as well as other features of a lack of secondary sexual characteristics, small testicles and gynaecomastia) can be found in patients with Klinefelter syndrome. Note that this patient is tall and obese.*
   (max. 2 marks)
2B. Intertrigo and/or fungal infections (1)
   Acanthosis nigricans (1) *on groins*
   Skin tags (1) *on groins*
   Striae distensae (1)
   Cellulite (0) *is very uncommon in men*
   (max. 2 marks)
3. Liver cirrhosis (1) from possibly chronic Hepatitis B infection (0.5) and/or non-alcoholic steatohepatitis (NASH) (0.5), which was contributed by diabetes and obesity (0.5).
   (max. 2 marks)
4. Likely reduced insulin degradation in liver cirrhosis (1)
5. Atrophied testicles (1)
   Any sign of ascites, e.g. shifting dullness, fluid wave and everted umbilicus (1)
   Inguinal hernia (1)

Caput medusae (1)

Splenomegaly (0.5) *is unlikely to be palpable due to this patient's morbid obesity*

Bruises (0.5) *are rarely found on the abdominal surface*

Hepatomegaly (0) *is unlikely to be palpable due to liver shrinkage from the cirrhotic process; furthermore, this patient has morbid obesity, which makes liver palpation virtually impossible.*

(max. 3 marks)

6A. Hepatitis B viral DNA load (1)

Prothrombin time (1)

Serum albumin (1)

Paracentesis (0) *is not indicated as it was mentioned in the stem that the additional abdominal examination did not reveal abnormalities.*

(max. 2 marks)

6B. Ultrasound liver (1)

Elastrographic assessment (1), e.g. Fibroscan

CT or MRI abdomen (0) — *this patient is unlikely to be able to physically fit into a CT (or) MRI scanning machine*

(max. 2 marks)

7. Hepatic encephalopathy (1) *precipitated by a surge in ammonia production from colonic bacterial catabolism of nitrogenous source* due to upper gastrointestinal bleeding likely from varices (1).

Septic encephalopathy (1) from secondary peritonitis (1) *of ascites due to portal hypertension and hypoalbuminaemia from decompensated liver failure.*

Hypovolaemic shock (1) from massive variceal bleeding (1)

Severe hypoglycaemia from poor intake (1) — *less likely given the clinical context*

(max. 4 marks)

4.2

1. Scaly (0.5) erythematous (0.5) circular/oval/annular (0.5) plaques (0.5)
2. D (2) — *the morphology and distribution of the rash are suggestive of psoriasis. An extensor predilection is the usual distribution.*
3. B (2) — *would be good to know if she is taking beta-blockers as these can induce or aggravate psoriasis.*
4. D (2) — *in a person with frequent contact with water and detergents, you may expect to see evidence of cumulative-insult irritant contact dermatitis viz. loss of cuticles and boggy proximal nailfolds, both of which are absent here. Dystrophy of nailplates does NOT immediately equate to fungal nail infection! Notice the scaly erythematous plaques surrounding the nailplates, which in conjunction with the preceding signs are compatible with psoriasis.*
5. Most common nail signs: pitting (0.5), onycholysis (0.5), subungual hyperkeratosis (0.5).
    Less common nail signs: oil drop sign (0.5), leukonychia (0.5), splinter haemorrhages (0.5).
    (max. 2 marks)
6A. (Psoriatic) Dactylitis (1)
    Psoriatic arthritis (0.5 — *not specific enough*)
    Gout (0). *Even though gout may very rarely present as a sausage-like swelling of the digit, this patient clearly has psoriatic plaques on her feet. In any case, podagra is way more common in gout!*
    (max. 1 mark)
6B. B (2) — *systemic corticosteroid is generally avoided, or it may precipitate a pustular conversion of the psoriasis.*
6C. A (1) — *spondyloarthropathy is a common cause*
7. E (2) — *a comprehensive evaluation of a psoriasis patient should include checking for its comorbidities viz. metabolic syndrome, uveitis, arthropathy, anxiety-depressive disorder.*

8A. *She has developed* erythroderma *(or "generalised exfoliative dermatitis"). The oedema and temperature dysregulation (shivering) are characteristics. It can be precipitated by a variety of causes:*
Noncompliance to therapy (1)
Her blood pressure medicine was changed to a beta-blocker (1)
Natural progression/extension of disease; unstable disease (1)
She was taking systemic corticosteroid from outside (1)
Other provoking factors, e.g. infection and severe stress (1)
Allergic reaction to another drug (1)
(max. 2 marks)

8B. Remove or treat provoking factors (1)
Maintain hydration and fluid balance (1)
Keep warm and monitor temperature (1)
Repair skin barrier (1)
Institute systemic treatment of psoriasis (1)
Hospitalisation (0.5)
Sedating antihistamines (0.5)
(max. 2 marks)

4.3

1A. Angina (1)
Any feature of congestive heart failure (1), e.g. orthopnea, paroxysmal nocturnal dyspnea

1B. Foamy urine (1)
Reduced urine output (1)

2. Displaced cardiac apex **and** a third heart sound (1) — *note that a third heart sound on its own can be found in healthy young persons, patients with severe volume overload, or a restrictive filling pattern accompanying substantial contractile dysfunction.*
Scrotal OR sacral OR facial OR scalp oedema (1) OR abdominal shifting dullness (1)
(max. 2 marks)

3.   Absence of Q waves to suggest old myocardial infarct (1)
     Absence of acute changes to suggest new or recent myocardial infarction (1)
     Voltage criteria for left ventricular hypertrophy to indicate hypertensive heart disease (1)
     Prolonged PR interval (0.5)
     (max. 2 marks)
4.   Elevated troponin T in the absence of chest pain and electrocardiographic changes is likely due to chronic kidney disease (1). *Trending the troponin T with clinical correlation is important. Postulated reasons for raised troponin T in chronic kidney disease (CKD) patients are microinfarctions, left ventricular hypertrophy, oxidative injury and reduced clearance.*
5.   24-hour urine total protein (1)
     Urine albumin: creatinine ratio (0)
     Repeat urine protein: creatinine ratio (0)
6.   **Nephrotic range** proteinuria (1) with **acute-on-chronic** kidney disease (1) presenting with volume overload (0.5)
     Chronic kidney disease (0.5)
     Acute kidney injury (0.5)
     Nephrotic syndrome (0)
     (max. 2 marks)
7.   Diabetic kidney disease (1) — *note evidence of diabetic microvascular changes of diabetic retinopathy*
     Hepatitis B related chronic glomerulonephritis (1) — *note the proteinuria and microscopic haematuria, positive HBsAg*
     Paraprotein related kidney disease (1), *e.g. multiple myeloma — note presence of anaemia and heavy proteinuria*
     Renal vein thrombosis (1) — *note the renal impairment, haematuria and proteinuria; not common but consider in patients with severe hypoalbuminaemia (serum albumin ≤ 20 g/dl).*
     (max. 2 marks)
8.   Ensure adequate blood pressure control (1)
     Ensure no coagulopathy (1)

Ensure that the patient fully understands the process (informed consent) and can cooperate with the procedure (1)
(max. 2 marks)

9. Optimal glycaemic control (1)
   Optimal blood pressure control (1) — *target ≤ 130/80 mmHg*
   Use of renin-angiotensin blockade (1)
   Avoidance of nephrotoxic agents (1)
   Evaluation of cardiovascular risks (1)
   (max. 2 marks)

10. Angiotensin II receptor blocker (1) *can cause the hyperkalaemia*
    Hyporeninemic hypoaldosteronism or type IV renal tubular acidosis (1) *can cause hyperkalaemia with normal anion gap metabolic acidosis*

4.4

1. Distal (1) muscle wasting (1)
   Foot drop (1) — if no mention of distal muscle wasting, only 0.5 marks. *Some patients who are in a very relaxed state may have their feet resting in a plantar flexed position at rest. Hence it is imperative to exclude the presence of foot drop by asking the patient to dorsiflex the feet.*
   (max. 2 marks)

2. Peripheral neuropathy (1)

3. Medication history (1)
   Dietary history (1)
   History of chronic alcohol consumption (1)
   (max. 2 marks)

4A. Pancytopenia (1)
    Macrocytosis (1)
    Raised mean corpuscular haemoglobin (MCH) (0.5)
    Increased RDW (0.5)
    (max. 2 marks)

4B. Megaloblastic anaemia (2)

Myelodysplastic disease OR primary marrow disease (2)

(max. 2 marks)

5. Haemolysis (suggested by the increased MCH) is a well-recognised phenomenon in B12 deficiency (1) *attributed to the intramedullary destruction of fragile cells from ineffective erythropoiesis*

6. Intrinsic factor antibody (1)

Evidence of haemolysis viz. LDH, indirect bilirubin, peripheral blood smear and reticulocyte count (1).

Fasting blood glucose (0.5) *would routinely be ordered in patients with peripheral neuropathy, but in this case, diabetes is not suspected.*

(max. 2 marks)

7. Avoidance of high cholesterol foodstuff (0.5)

Malnutrition (1)

Malignancy (1)

(max. 2 marks)

Low cholesterol may be due to inherited causes or acquired disease. Multiple diseases have been associated with low cholesterol or low-density lipoprotein (LDL), and these include patients with carcinoma, multiple myeloma, severe illness, malabsorption or pernicious anaemia, or nutritional deficiencies. Studies have shown vegans generally have lower LDLs and higher high-density lipoproteins (HDLs). Those who avoid meat may also have low cholesterol levels. Trans fats are added to processed foods for longer shelf life and may elevate cholesterols in those who take processed food.

8. Subacute combined degeneration of the cord (2) *as evidenced by the combined presence of gait problems, peripheral neuropathy and B12 deficiency.*

9. Shades areas covered by A (1), *which are responsible for loss of proprioception*

Shades areas covered by B (1), *which are responsible for weakness*

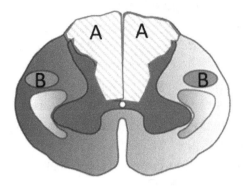

10. Limb hypertonia (1)
    Loss of vibration sense (1)
    Positive Romberg's test (1)
    Gait disturbances (0.5) — *e.g. ataxic, stamping*
    (max. 2 marks)

4.5

1. Reflex syncope (1), *e.g. vasovagal syncope, situational syncope, carotid sinus syncope; and*
   Orthostatic hypotension (1) *are universally very common causes of syncope across all ages.*
   Cardiogenic syncope (1), *e.g. structural cardiac disease, and arrhythmia (as she is taking atenolol, consider the possibility of a bradyarrhythmia) is a particularly important cause in the elderly. Furthermore, irradiation in the neck can affect the functionality of baroreceptors, causing recurrent syncope.*
   Vertebrobasilar transient ischaemic attack (1) *and*
   Subclavian steal syndrome (1) *may be considered as she has an atherosclerotic risk.*

Hypoglycaemia (0.5) *is possible in a diabetic person, especially in the elderly, but the risk is generally low with metformin and a dipeptidyl peptidase 4 (DPP4) inhibitor like linagliptin.*

Epilepsy (0) *should be considered in the absence of the above syncopal causes and in the presence of observed seizures. In contrast to syncope, epilepsy usually gives a longer period of unconsciousness. Also. note that small-vessel strokes such as a lacunar stroke do not usually cause scarring epilepsy.*

(max. 4 marks)

2. Postural blood pressure measurement (1)
    Electrocardiogram (ECG) (1)
    Capillary blood glucose (0)
    Carotid sinus massage (0) *should not be performed in someone who has had a recent stroke. Additionally, it may further cause bradycardia due to a high vagal tone.*

3A. Orthostatic hypotension (1)

3B. High dose of Prazocin (1). *Any antihypertensive medication can potentially cause or exacerbate orthostatic hypotension, but in this context, this very potent α-1 adrenergic antagonist stands out as the most likely drug culprit.*

    Combined effects of antihypertensive medications (1)
    Autonomic dysfunction secondary to poorly-controlled diabetes (1)
    Autonomic dysfunction in the elderly (0) *may be considered only after ruling out obvious reversible causes such as the above.*

    Addison's disease or hypoadrenalism (0) *should not be considered at this stage given the lack of compatible history, physical findings and biochemistry.*

    (max. 2 marks)

4. Low levels of basal serum cortisol (0.5) and ACTH (0.5)
    Inadequate serum cortisol response to ACTH (Synacthen) (1)
    — *less than 500 nmol/L.*
    Suggestive of secondary adrenal insufficiency (1)

5A. Central hypothyroidism (1)

5B. Hypopituitarism (1)
Due to previous neck irradiation (1)
For nasopharyngeal carcinoma (1)

6. D (1)

7. C (1) — *in a patient with both hypothyroidism and adrenal insufficiency, thyroxine replacement should not be administered until the adrenal insufficiency is adequately treated. Treating hypothyroidism alone may increase the clearance of the little cortisol that is produced, therefore worsening the cortisol deficiency.*

8. Hypothyroidism (1)
History of radiation therapy for nasopharyngeal carcinoma (NPC) (1)
Senescence (1)
Drug-induced (0) — *none of her drugs is known to be ototoxic*
(max. 2 marks)

Assessment Paper 5

5.1

1. Duputyren's contracture (1)
Leukonychia (1) *totalis*
Clubbing (0) *cannot be determined at this view*

2. Asterixis (1)
Finger clubbing (1)
Wasting of intrinsic muscles of the hand (1) — *indicative of peripheral neuropathy*
Tar stains (0.5) — *may be evident in a chronic smoker but not particularly contributory*

Palmar erythema (0) — *it is clearly not present here*
(max. 2 marks)

3.   Alcohol intoxication (1)
Hepatic encephalopathy (1)
Wernicke-Korsakoff syndrome (1) — *due to dry beriberi*
Head injury (1)
Meningitis (1)
Hypoglycaemia (1)
Stroke (0) *would have focal neurology. Blood pressure is often high in subarachnoid haemorrhage. If the stroke is confined to the cerebellum his conscious state should be intact.*
(max. 3 marks)

4.   Chronic alcohol intake (1)
Chronic liver disease (1)
Drug-related (1) — *e.g. azathioprine, methotrexate*
Reticulocytosis (1) *as it is likely he has had gastrointestinal bleeding before as well*
Hypothyroidism (0.5) *is a cause of macrocytosis but there is no clinical feature to suggest it so far*
Vitamin B12 and/or folate deficiency (0) — *will give megaboblastic macrocytosis!*
(max. 2 marks)

5.   A, D, F and G (1 × 4 = 4 marks). *Terlipressin is better than somatostatin/octreotide for acute variceal bleeding. Ceftriaxone prevents bacterial translocation in variceal bleed and also treats bacterial meningitis. It is important to administer thiamine prior to or simultaneously with glucose (if hypoglycaemic) in an alcohol-intoxicated patient.*

6A. Red cell transketolase level (1)
Blood sugar level (1)
Blood alcohol level (1)
(max. 2 marks)

6B. An electroencephalogram (EEG) (1) *to differentiate alcohol intoxication, hepatic encephalopathy, etc.*

CT/MRI brain scan (1)

Lumbar puncture (1) *for meningitis*

(max. 2 marks)

7. ***The aim is to prevent hepatic encephalopathy, Wernicke-Korsakoff syndrome and variceal bleed:***

Lactulose (1)

Thiamine (1)

Propranolol (1)

Repeated banding of oesophageal varices until they are obliterated (1)

Alcohol cessation (1)

(max. 3 marks)

5.2

1. Ischaemic optic neuropathy (1)

Optic neuritis (1)

Migraine (1)

All these conditions are painless (0): retinal detachment, central retinal artery or vein occlusion, vitreous haemorrhage.

All these conditions have redness (0): acute glaucoma, bacterial or viral keratitis, anterior uveitis, endopthalmitis.

(max. 2 marks)

2. A (2) — a *CT brain scan to evaluate the cause of intracranial pressure should be ordered stat.*

3. Glasgow Coma Scale (GCS) score (1)

Blood pressure and pulse rate (1) *to watch for Cushing's response*

Pupillary changes (1)

Impaired extraocular movements (1)

Monitoring for spreading of haemorrhage over external eye (1) — *important sign of cavernous sinus thrombosis*

(max. 3 marks)

4. Increased intracranial pressure *(false localising sign of new 6th nerve palsy)* (1)
    Mononeuritis due to diabetes (0.5)
    (max. 1 mark)
5. History of venous clotting events (1)
    History of miscarriages (1)
    History of usage of oral contraceptive pill (1)
    Family history of clotting disorders OR autoimmune disease (1)
    Unexplained weight loss (1)
    History of breast lumps or nipple discharge OR unexplained systemic symptoms (1)
    Symptoms of autoimmune disease (e.g. oral ulcers, joint pains, photosensitivity, alopecia) (1)
    (max. 4 marks)
6A. Lupus anticoagulant OR Anti-cardiolipin antibodies (1)
    PLUS
    ANA (0.5)
    Anti-dsDNA (0.5)
    Homocysteine (0.5)
    (max 1 mark)
    Protein C, Protein S, Anti-thrombin III (0) *can be low in an acute phase of thrombosis, so these should be checked at a later date.*
6B. JAK2 mutation — *should be considered even if the full blood count was normal as cerebral venous thrombosis may precede the development of myeloproliferative conditions.*
6C. Mammogram (1)
    CT scan of the thorax, abdomen and pelvis (OR PET-CT) (1)
    Ultrasound thyroid gland (1)
    (max. 2 marks)
7. Thyroid-stimulating hormone OR Thyroid function test (2) — *hypothyroidism, if inadequately treated, is an important cause of menorrhagia!*

5.3

1A. Protopsis (1) OR Exopthalmos (1)
Mild left upper lid oedema (0.5)
(max. 1 mark)

1B. Conjunctival suffusion OR keratoconjunctivitis (1)
Corneal ulceration (1)
(max. 1 mark)

2. Diffuse (1) enlargement
Thrill (1)
Warmth (1)
Tenderness (0)
Bruit (0) *is an auscultatory finding not on palpation. It is almost always present, especially if you can feel a thrill.*
(max. 2 marks)

3. Palmar erythema (0.5)
Hyperhidrosis (0.5)
Action tremor (0.5)
Finger clubbing (plus soft tissue swelling of fingers equates to thyroid acropachy) ($0.5 \times 2 = 1$ mark)
Onycholysis (Plummer's nails) (0.5)
(max. 2 marks)

4. Thyroid-stimulating hormone (TSH) receptor antibody (1) *is suggestive of Graves' disease.*

5. Full blood count (1) — *thionamides are contraindicated if the absolute neutrophil count is low*
Liver function test (1) — *thionamides are contraindicated in severe liver derangement*

6. Smoking cessation (2) *has been shown to reduce the severity of Graves' disease and Graves' orbitopathy*
Avoidance of excessive dietary iodine (1)
Stress management (1) *is important but not the most crucial non-pharmacological treatment here*
(max. 2 marks)

7. Pericardial rub (1) *due to thyrotoxic pericarditis*
    Means–Lerman scratch (1) *due to rubbing of the hyperdynamic pericardium against the pleura*
    (max. 1 mark)
8. Bounding pulse (0.5)
    Irregularly irregular pulse/heart rate (0.5)
    Hypertension (0.5)
    Feature(s) of heart failure, e.g. basal crepitations, elevated jugular venous pressure, peripheral oedema (max. 1 mark)
    (max. 2 marks)
9A. Absent p waves (0.5)
    Irregular ventricular rate (0.5)
9B. B (2)
10. Carbimazole-induced *(ANCA-positive)* vasculitis (1)
    Henoch-Schonlein purpura (0)
11. Thyroidectomy (1) as Graves' orbitopathy can be resistant to medical treatment (1)
    Radioactive iodine (0) *can aggravate Graves' orbitopathy.*

5.4

1. High anion gap metabolic acidosis (1)
2. Salicylate level (1)
    Paracetamol level (1)
    Serum lactic acid level (1) — *can be elevated in ethylene glycol and methanol poisoning, but it is often mild, and the degree of acidosis is disproportional to the level of serum lactate.*
    Venous blood gas (1) — *this is to look for pH and CO_2, **only** in this setting whereby time is of essence*
    Serum osmolality and/or osmolal gap (0.5) — *Presence of a large osmolal gap (the difference between calculated and measured osmolality) of >10 mOsm/kg indicates the presence*

of an osmotically active, electrically neutral substance like alcohol but it will not help you differentiate one from the other. The key differentiating features between the less toxic ethanol, isopropyl alcohol and the more toxic methanol and ethylene glycol is the severe high anion gap metabolic acidosis (HAGMA) present with the latter.

Blood alcohol level (0.5) — *the key limitation of the test is that the blood is usually sent to reference laboratories, and the turnaround time of "sent out" tests is usually long. In such an acute situation of suspected poisoning where early diagnosis and treatment are crucial in terms of preventing the risk of sequelae, one often cannot wait for the result to make management decisions.*

Procalcitonin level (0.5) — *one would have expected a higher grade of fever in sepsis*

Cardiac enzymes (0)

(max. 3 marks)

3. D (2) — *"do not resuscitate" orders and "advance care planning" documents are meant to ensure that the patient receives appropriate care. The patient's and his family's wishes are taken into consideration but the final decision should come from the medical team who acts in the best interest of the patient. These are not legally binding documents and can be changed if necessary based on the circumstances. In this situation, the patient is likely to have an easily reversible condition with a high chance of recovery if he is managed in the intensive care unit (ICU). As the incident happened in the hospital, which was captured by CCTV, it confers a reasonable degree of certainty to the medical team about the amount and content consumed by the patient and the chance of achieving a successful outcome with treatment. Moreover, as the hospital is responsible for preventing this act while the patient is hospitalised, this case has the potential to become a medicolegal and media case. Bearing all these in mind, his extent of care and*

resuscitation decision was reversed after discussion with the family and he was transferred to the ICU.

4A. Osmolol gap = serum osmolality − calculated serum osmolality
= 374 − [2(142) + 13.2 + 16.2] = 60.6 (1)
Is significantly increased (1)
Indicates the presence of an osmotically active electrically neutral substance, e.g. alcohol (1)
(max. 2 marks)

4B. Ketosis (0.5) is likely due to alcohol toxicity (1) rather than diabetes (0.5), *as ketones and glucose levels were normal in the first set of blood. Isopropyl alcohol is metabolised to acetone by alcohol dehydrogenase. As a result, ketones will be strongly positive in blood and urine two hours after ingestion.*

4C. Tissue hypoxia (1) *due to shock*
Vitamin B1 deficiency (1) *causing a deficiency in pyruvate dehydrogenase. Note that this patient is prone to Vitamin B1 deficiency as he had a history of chronic alcoholism and his nutrition state is unknown. Beriberi can mimic severe sepsis-like syndrome with shock, severe HAGMA and multiorgan failure, which can often be life-threatening!*
Toxins, e.g. ethanol, ethylene glycol, methanol (1)
Lactic acidosis due to metformin (0.5)
Inborn errors of metabolism (0)
(max. 2 marks)

4D. Acute kidney impairment (1)
False positive elevation in creatinine due to acetone generated from the metabolism of isopropyl alcohol (1)

4E. Urine microscopy revealing calcium oxalate crystals gives a clue to the diagnosis of ethylene glycol in the relevant clinical setting, but **the absence of these crystals does not rule out ethylene glycol poisoning** as it takes a few hours for these crystals to form. (1)

5. Mixed metabolic and respiratory acidosis (2) — *primarily severe metabolic acidosis causing cardiopulmonary collapse, which contributes to respiratory acidosis.*

6. *Like ethanol, which competitively inhibits alcohol dehydrogenase, fomepizole is useful in methanol and ethylene glycol poisoning as it prevents the generation of toxic metabolites that cause organ failure.* The primary metabolite of isopropyl alcohol is acetone, and it is less toxic than isopropyl alcohol itself, thus there is no indication for inhibition of alcohol dehydrogenase in this setting. (1)

7. A (2) — *the use of frusemide to prevent or postpone dialysis is not recommended by any guideline. Continuous renal replacement therapy is the most ideal as the patient is haemodynamically unstable and on inotropic support. Haemodialysis is rarely required for isopropyl alcohol poisoning; it is very effective in the setting of methanol and ethylene glycol poisoning with acidosis and end-organ dysfunction and should be considered even if the renal function is normal.*

5.5

1. Acute viral infection (1), *e.g. dengue, HIV, EBV, human parvovirus B19*
   Reactive arthritis (1) — *this is a form of arthritis developing soon after or during an infection elsewhere in the body, but in which the micro-organism does not enter the joint.*
   Septic arthritis (nongonococcal or gonococcal arthritis) (1)
   Acute lupus (0.5) — *fever is a common but non-specific symptom of systemic lupus erythematosus (SLE), and the temperature spikes are rarely markedly high such as the case in this patient.*

Crystal-related arthritis (0.5) — *this is rare in women of her age, and even less likely without any other risk factors*
Serum sickness (0) — *the "latent period" is too long here*
(max. 2 marks)

2A. Temperature spiking twice daily ("double quotidian fever") (1)
Each spike is marked (>39°C) (0.5) and lasts for few hours (0.5)
Temperature returns to normal or below normal between fever spikes (1)
(max. 2 marks)

2B. Adult-onset Still's Disease (AOSD) (1)
(Mixed) malarial infections (1)
Kala-azar OR Visceral leishmaniasis (1)
Miliary tuberculosis (1)
Legionellosis (1)
Kawasaki disease (0) *is a paediatric condition*
Infective endocarditis (0) *typically has either remittent or continuous fever*
(max. 2 marks)

3A. Dropped likely due to acute infection. *In acute infections, complement opsonised particles bind to the complement receptor 1 on red blood cells (RBCs), which are transported to the spleen and liver. There, they are removed by residential macrophages* (1).

3B. Neutrophilic leukocytosis can have many causes, e.g. bacterial infections, systemic inflammatory diseases, tissue hypoxia stimulating neutrophil release from marrow, etc. (1)

3C. Thrombocytosis most likely reactive to acute infection or systemic inflammation (1)

3D. Mild transaminitis (<5x above upper limit) may signify viral hepatitis, non-alcoholic steatohepatitis, autoimmune hepatitis, toxic or drug-induced hepatitis (1).

4. Full blood count (1)
C-reactive protein OR procalcitonin (1)

Liver panel (1)

Repeat blood culture (1)

CT abdomen/pelvis scan (1) — *to look for the source of infection*

Transthoracic echocardiography (1) — *to look for the source of infection*

Serum ferritin (1)

Viral hepatitis serology (0.5) — *can be considered if the liver enzymes continue to escalate, though viral hepatitis would not have caused neutrophilic leukocytosis.*

Left knee aspiration for microscopy, cell count and culture (0.5) – *the effusion was described as "small"*

Autoimmune serologies to evaluate for connective tissue disease (CTD)/SLE (such as ANA and anti-dsDNA) (0) — *very unlikely at this point, especially in the context of leukocytosis and thrombocytosis*

Joint X-rays (0)

The erythrocyte sedimentation rate (ESR) (0) *is inferior to c-reactive protein (CRP) or procalcitonin when monitoring for progress/deterioration in acute inflammation/sepsis.*

Urine culture (0)

Bone marrow biopsy (0)

(max. 4 marks)

5. AOSD (2) — *extreme hyperferritinaemia (> 10,000 ug/L) in conjunction with pyrexia of unknown origin should point to either AOSD or haemophagocytic lymphohistiocytosis.*

    Haemochromatosis (0) *does not present with pyrexia of unknown origin*

6. Systemic corticosteroid (2) *in doses equivalent to prednisolone 1 mg/kg/day for a patient with moderate disease characterised by high fever, polyarthritis and mild internal organ involvement.*

Oral nonsteroidal anti-inflammatory drugs (NSAIDs) (1) *may be used in mild diseases presenting with fever, rash and arthralgia.*
Extend coverage of broad-spectrum antibiotic (0)
(max. 2 marks)

7. Macrophage activation syndrome (MAS) (1) — *secondary (reactive) haemophagocytic syndrome occurring in 5–12% of AOSD patients*

8. Consumptive coagulopathy (1) — *there is evidence of disseminated intravascular coagulation with elevated PT/APTT and causing low fibrinogen level.*

Assessment Paper 6

6.1

1. A (2) — *must auscultate the chest for small airway obstruction; this is especially critical given that this tachypnoeic patient is saturating at 92% on room air!*

2A. E (1) — *annular confluent oedematous-erythematous plaques*

2B. D (1) — *annular erythematous plaques with scaly periphery and central clearing*

3A. A (2) — *all interventions are important, but the top priority is adrenaline!*

3B. IM (0.5) adrenaline 1:1000 (0.5) 0.3–0.5 mg (0.5) over antero-lateral thigh (0.5) — *this is one of the few drugs that you ought to know the precise dose and route as it is life-saving!*

4. A (2) — *do not worry about repeating adrenaline in severe anaphylaxis if response is suboptimal at five minutes. This is life-saving!*

5. D (2) — *tryptase is a mast cell-released mediator and is elevated in anaphylaxis. So too is histamine, but it peaks within 5–10 minutes of symptom onset and normalises within 15–30 minutes, whereas tryptase has a longer half-life. It is generally recommended that three samples be taken as soon as possible, after 1–2 hours, and after 24 hours of symptom onset.*

6. A and C (1 × 2 = 2 marks) — *apart from a young age and a background of asthma, other risk multipliers include a past history of severe reaction, the patient taking a beta blocker or an ACEI (or both), late or absent treatment initiation, and a history of systemic mastocytosis.*

7. A (2) — *the patient should be observed for a biphasic reaction. The period of observation ranges from 1 to 24 hours after symptom resolution of the index reaction.*

8. Referral to allergist (1)

   Avoidance of any nonsteroidal anti-inflammatory drugs (NSAID) (1) including diclofenac (0.5)

   Information about anaphylaxis (1)

   Drug allergy card (1)

   (max. 4 marks)

6.2

1. Fundoscopy (1) to look for papiloedema (0.5), which indicates raised intracranial pressure (0.5).

   > **PLUS**
   >
   > Otoscopy (1) to look for otitis media (0.5), which could have led to meningitis (0.5).
   >
   > Oral mucosal examination (1) to look for clinical dehydration (0.5) from vomiting and poor intake (0.5)

Cranial VI nerve palsy (1), which indicates increased intracranial pressure (0.5) due to meningitis (0.5).
Sensorineural hearing loss (1), which suggests *Streptococcus suis* meningitis (1).
Eschar (1), which suggests typhus meningitis (1).
(max. 2 marks)

2. Acute meningitis (1)

3A. *Streptococcus pneumoniae* (1)
Group B Streptococcus (1)
Haemophilus influenzae (1)
Ricketssiae sp (0.5) — *not as common as the others*
(max. 2 marks)

3B. Herpes Simplex (1)
Treponema pallidum (1)
(max. 2 marks)

4. Intravenous hydration (1)
Immediate lumbar puncture (1)
Immediate droplet isolation (1)
Close monitoring (1)
CT brain scan (0) — *the patient did not fulfil the Infectious Diseases Society of America (ISDA) criteria for needing a CT brain scan viz. a seizure, papiloedema (it was mentioned in the question that the additional physical examination, which should include a fundoscopy, was unremarkable), an immunocompromised host, depressed GCS, and an age of more than 60 years.*
(max. 3 marks)

5. Dexamethasone (1)
Ceftriaxone (1)
Vancomycin (1)
Acyclovir (1)

6. All his room-mates (1) should be given prophylactic ciprofloxacin/rifampicin (1)

7. Complement studies (1)
   Immunoglobulin levels (1)
   In a patient with recurrent meningococcaemia, remember to look closely for a splenectomy scar!

6.3

1. Sinus tachycardia (1)
   S1Q3T3 pattern in an electrocardiogram (ECG) (1)
   Observation on chest X-ray (0)
2. Pulmonary embolism (1)
   Acute myocardial infarction (1)— *inferior OR right ventricular*
3. Pulseless electrical activity (1)
4. Intravenous fluids (1)
   Inotropic support (0.5) *may be needed if fluid resuscitation is not sufficient to stabilise the blood pressure*
   (max. 1 mark)
5. B (2)
6. D (2) — *if the 2Decho shows signs of severe right heart strain, thin RV walls, D-shaped septum, it can be adequate evidence for an acute right heart obstruction event, which can be either a pneumothorax or pulmonary embolism.*
7. Hypoxaemia (0.5) and respiratory alkalosis (0.5) with incomplete (0.5) metabolic compensation (0.5)
8. Increase FiO_2 on the ventilator (1)
   Give sodium bicarbonate (0)
   Increase sedation (0)
9. Packed cell transfusion (1) *x2 packs*
   Fresh frozen plasma (1) *x500 ml*
   Intravenous (0.5) Vitamin K (0.5) — *10 mg*

Arrange for oesophagogastroduodenoscopy (1)

Intravenous (0.5) proton-pump inhibitor (0.5)

Keep nil by mouth and set intravenous drip (0) *are essential actions but not strictly "therapeutic"*

(max. 4 marks)

10. Warn that omeprazole can potentiate the effect of warfarin (1)
Attend all sessions with the physician or pharmacist on INR testing and dose adjustments (1)

Watch for easy bruising and inform the physician or pharmacist (1)

Avoid food or drugs that further increase the risk of bleeding (1), *e.g. nonsteroidal anti-inflammatory drugs, certain antibiotics, excess alcohol, grapefruit juice.*

(max. 3 marks)

6.4

1. Postural hypotension (1) *due to diabetic autonomic neuropathy, possible adrenal insufficiency*

Impaired vision (1) *due to diabetic retinopathy or cataracts*

Peripheral neuropathy (1) *due to poor diabetic control*

Musculoskeletal causes (1) *such as rheumatoid arthritic flare and joint deformities*

Vertebrobasilar insufficiency (1) *with risk factors of age, diabetes and atherosclerosis*

Anaemia (1), *as this is an elderly with light-headedness and risk factors of age, diabetes and rheumatoid arthritis*

(max. 4 marks)

2A. Adrenal insufficiency (1) — *secondary to long-term steroids*

Chronic kidney disease (1) — *impairs free water excretion*

Syndrome of inappropriate ADH secretion (SIADH) (0) — *indeed, this may occur due to a head injury after falls, but it cannot be considered at this stage as the renal function is impaired and other causes of hyponatraemia have not yet been excluded. Classically in SIADH, urea, creatinine, sodium and chloride are all low.*

2B. Short Synacthen test OR 8 am Cortisol (1) — *note that 8 am Cortisol is only useful if the absolute value is less than 100 nmol/L, otherwise its diagnostic utility is low, a very common misconception!*

Thyroid function test (1)

Plasma and urine osmolalities (1)

24-hour creatinine clearance test (1)

(max. 2 marks)

3A. Osteoporosis (1)

3B. Rheumatoid arthritis (1)

Post-menopausal (1)

Lack of weight bearing activities (1)

Long-term use of steroid (1)

The following risk factors were absent from the history:

Dietary lack of calcium (0.5)

Low weight (0.5)

Family history of osteoporosis (0.5)

Smoking (0.5)

Alcohol intake (0.5)

(max. 4 marks)

3C. Fracture Risk Assessment tool (FRAX) (1)

4. E (1) — *one glass of milk only confers about 300 mg of calcium; about 1,200 mg calcium daily is needed for good bone health in the elderly.*

5. A (1) — *apart from bisphosphonates and calcium/Vitamin D supplementation, other viable options are denosumab, selective oestrogen receptor modulators (SERMs), teriparatide and strontium. Calcitonin is mainly given to people with acute osteoporotic vertebral fractures. The place of oral magnesium is currently not widely accepted. Oestrogen-progestin is now no longer considered as first-line therapy given the presence of multiple good alternative*

anti-osteoporotic drugs, and the risks of coronary artery disease, stroke, breast cancer and venous thromboembolism.

6. Synovial thickening (1)
    Degenerative changes (0.5)

7. Anaemia of chronic disease (1) *(rheumatoid arthritis and diabetic nephropathy)*
    Bone marrow suppression (1) *from immunosuppressive medication, e.g. methotrexate*
    Gastrointestinal bleeding (1) *from nonsteroidal anti-inflammatory drugs and corticosteroids*
    Felty syndrome (1) — *a rare association with seropositive rheumatoid arthritis*
    Megaloblastic anaemia (1) *(folate deficiency due to methotrexate for rheumatoid arthritis; Vitamin B12 deficiency due to pernicious anaemia, which is infrequently associated with rheumatoid arthritis).*
    (max. 3 marks)

6.5

1. One of the most common causes of delayed puberty is a transient functional defect in the production of gonadotrophin-releasing hormones (GnRH) from the hypothalamus, and this may be due to physiological variation that can be genetic (1). *Hence, children of parents with delayed puberty may also have delayed puberty. Note that even Kallman syndrome/hypogonadotrophic hypogonadism can be familial.*

2. Anosmia/Hyposmia and colour blindness are associated with Kallman syndrome (isolated gonadotropin deficiency) (1)
    Visual field problems may be associated with hypothalamic-pituitary disorders (1)

3. Tall stature suggests normal growth hormone dynamics. The growth hormone may be affected in hypothalamic-pituitary

disorders and is unaffected if there is pure isolated GnRH deficiency, which can be congenital (2).

4. Klinefelter syndrome OR Hypogonadotrophic hypogonadism (1)
5. Absent or sparse axillary, pubic or facial (beard) hair (1)
    Under-developed limb musculature (1)
    Under-development of external genitalia (1), *e.g. micropenis, hypospadias, cryptochidism*
    Speech and language deficits (0.5)
    Broad hips (0) — *is already implied by "centripetal obesity" in the stem*
    Lower segment measuring more than the upper segment; arms span measuring greater than the height (0) *are features already implied by "eunuchoid habitus" in the stem.*
    (max. 2 marks)
6. D (2) — *the hormonal assay suggests hypogonadotrophic hypogonadism*
7. Full blood count (FBC) (1)
    Prostate specific antigen (1)
    Patients receiving testosterone should be monitored clinically (symptoms of androgenisation and in terms of libido). It is standard to monitor their FBC and prostate-specific antigen (PSA) as testosterone stimulates erythropoiesis and causes prostatic hypertrophy.
    Testosterone level (0.5). *Some physicians prefer to measure testosterone levels midway between injections to achieve the optimal levels.*
    (max. 2 marks)
8. History of chronic smoking (0.5) as it can cause polycythaemia for many reasons (0.5), *including hypoxia, carbon monoxide exposure, smoking-related disease and volume contraction.*
    PLUS
    The history of snoring/daytime somnolence (0.5) is suggestive of obstructive sleep apnoea, which is a hypoxic state (0.5) *that can stimulate erythropoiesis.*

Headaches/fatigue/blurred vision/paraesthesia (0.5) are all symptoms of hyper-viscosity syndrome (0.5) *in polycythaemia*

Acute episodes of joint pain/painful swelling of the big toe (0.5) suggest gout (0.5), *which can occur due to increased cellular turnover in polycythaemia*

(max. 1 mark)

9. Splenomegaly (0.5) frequently occurs in polycythaemia vera (PV) OR myeloproliferative disease (0.5).

   PLUS

   Gouty tophi (0.5) may be a complication of PV (0.5)

   Hypertension (0.5), usually mild, can be seen in PRV (0.5). *Note that hypertension may also suggest phaeo-chromocytoma, a rare cause of secondary polycythaemia.*

   Bruises (0.5) can be due to bleeding tendency (0.5) *in PV*

   Ballotable kidney (0.5) may suggest a renal tumour, polycystic kidney (0.5), *which are secondary causes of polycythaemia.*

   Any clinical sign of dehydration (0.5), which may indicate relative polycythaemia (0.5).

   Cerebellar signs (0.5), which may suggest cerebellar haemangioblastoma (0.5), is an extremely rare cause of secondary polycythaemia.

   (max. 1 mark)

10. Urine microscopy (1) — *haematuria may occur in renal tumours or cysts*

    Serum erythropoetin level (1) — *erythropoietin levels are low in PV; high erythropoietin levels occur in tumours producing erythropoietin or in reactive states, which cause polycythaemia.*

    Serum JAK2 mutation (1) — *more than 95% of patients with PV have a positive JAK2 mutation*

    (max. 2 marks)

11. Testosterone replacement was temporarily suspended OR the patient defaulted on his injections (1)
Testosterone dose was attenuated (1)
Intervals between testosterone injections were increased (1) (max. 2 marks)
[Where testosterone is responsible for the polycythaemia, particularly when haematocrit is above 54%, testosterone cessation is recommended. Where the haematocrit percentage drops, then testosterone can be restarted at lower doses or with increased intervals between injections. This man's dose was slightly reduced, and the interval increased to optimise the haemoglobin and haematocrit.]

Assessment Paper 7

7.1

1. Hypertensive heart disease (1)
Ischaemic heart disease (1). *She may have a previous silent or missed coronary event.*
Cardiomyopathy due to obesity (1) *and obstructive sleep apnoea*
Rheumatic heart disease (0) *may uncommonly present at this age with heart failure due to valvular dysfunction but is usually characterised by cardiac murmur(s).*
2. C (2) — *diuretic usually improves congestion and symptoms and signs of heart failure. For those on chronic diuretic therapy, an initial IV dose should be at least equivalent to an oral dose. Immediate echocardiography is recommended if cardiogenic shock is suspected.*

3. Left ventricular hypertrophy (1)
   Minimal ST depression in V6 (1) — *suggestive of strain (hypertensive heart disease)*
   Sinus tachycardia (1)
   (max. 2 marks)

4. Upper lobe diversion OR dilatation of upper lobe pulmonary veins (1)
   Perihilar alveolar oedema OR peribronchial cuffing (1)
   Cardiomegaly (1) *as cardiothoracic ratio > 0.50*
   Kerley B lines (0) — *not seen here*
   (max. 2 marks)

5. NT-proBNP (0.5)
   FBC (0.5)
   Urea and electrolytes (0.5) with estimated GFR (0.5)
   Liver function (0.5)
   Fasting blood glucose OR HbA1c (0.5)
   Cardiac enzymes OR Troponins (0.5)
   Fasting lipid panel (0.5)
   (max. 3 marks)

6. Heart failure with preserved ejection fraction (*HFpEF*) OR diastolic heart failure (1) because she has signs and symptoms of heart failure (0.5), normal systolic left ventricular function OR left ventricular ejection fraction (LVEF) > 50% (0.5), and the presence of a structural abnormality OR concentric left ventricular hypertrophy (0.5). Her risk factors for the development of this condition are female gender (0.5), older age (0.5), longstanding hypertension (0.5) and obesity (0.5).
   (max. 3 marks)

7. B (1) — *no treatment has yet been shown to reduce morbidity and mortality in patients with HFpEF. An important aim of treatment is to alleviate symptoms and improve well-being.*

8. D (2) — *diuretics, angiotensin converting enzyme (ACE) inhibitors, angiotensin II receptor blockers (ARBs), and mineralocorticoid receptor antagonists are appropriate agents,*

though a beta-blocker may be less effective in reducing systolic blood pressure. In particular, ACE inhibitors and ARBs have generally shown reductions in morbidity and hence play an important role in the treatment of the disease processes (hypertension, hypertensive heart disease, diabetes, chronic kidney disease) that contribute to the development of HFpEF.

9. B (2) — *ACE inhibitor-associated angioedema is related to bradykinin excess; thus antihistamines and corticosteroid are not useful. She does not appear to require airway protection at this stage.*

10. E (1) — *angioedema secondary to ACE inhibitors can occur at any point in time during its usage, not necessarily at the time of initiation. Re-challenge is absolutely not warranted. An ARB may be considered in place of an ACE inhibitor a few weeks after discontinuation.*

7.2

1. Chronic obstructive pulmonary disease (1)
Bronchial asthma (1)
Ischaemic heart disease (1)
Bronchiectasis (0.5)
Lung cancer (0.5)
Cor pulmonale (0.5)
(max. 3 marks)

2. Chronic obstructive pulmonary disease (1)
"Scooped out" appearance of the expiratory limb of the flow-volume loop (1)
FEV1/FVC ratio < 70% (1), *which confirms the presence of obstructive lung disease.*
Radiologic hyperinflation of lungs (1), *as evidenced by the presence of ten posterior ribs in the midclavicular line, and a (partial) flattening of the diaphragm.*
(max. 3 marks)

3.   B and F ($1 \times 2 = 2$ marks) — *arterial blood gas is not indicated when the patient has normal oxygen saturation; it will not help diagnose asthma or chronic obstructive pulmonary disease (COPD). Diffusion capacity evaluates for the presence of parenchymal lung disease if spirometry indicates a restrictive pattern. An electrocardiogram (ECG) may be helpful in the consideration of cardiac causes of breathlessness. Anaemia may aggravate breathlessness in a patient with chronic lung disease.*

4.   Smoking cessation counselling (1) *is the most important dis-ease-modifying treatment for COPD.*

     Long-acting β-agonist OR long-acting muscarinic antagonist (1) *is the mainstay of COPD pharmacotherapy.*

     Pulmonary rehabilitation (1) *has been shown to reduce symp-toms and improve exercise tolerance in all symptomatic COPD patients.*

     Inhaled corticosteroid (0) *is used as an* **add-on** *therapy for patients with frequent exacerbations despite inhaled bronchodilators.*

     Long-term oxygen therapy (0) *is only indicated for patients who are hypoxic (PaO_2 <55 mmHg at rest or <60 mmHg with complications, e.g. pulmonary hypertension).*

     Evaluation and management for cardiac causes (0) *may be con-sidered if the patient remains persistently dyspnoeic despite optimising COPD treatment.*

5.   Acute exacerbation of COPD (1)

     Acute myocardial infarction (1)

     Pneumothorax (1)

     Aortic dissection (0) — *would not explain the respiratory findings*

6.   B (1) — *the immediate priority is to correct the hypoxia, not performing further investigations. However, oxygen therapy should be titrated in COPD patients to target an oxygen*

saturation level of 88 to 92%. High-flow oxygen can worsen hypercapnia in patients who are chronic CO_2 retainers! Intubation is appropriate if the patient is comatose at presentation or failed to respond to initial therapy, or if the patient is confused and very hypoxaemic. The high blood pressure is not the primary problem — it is reactive to the acute respiratory distress that the patient was experiencing.

7. Acute respiratory acidosis (1). *Note that hypercapnia per se is not a diagnostic criterion for COPD — about 1 in 4 COPD patients have elevated $PaCO_2$ on their arterial blood gas!*

8. Nebulisation with short-acting bronchodilators (1) *to reduce bronchospasm*

   Non-invasive ventilation (1) *has morbidity (reduce intubation rate and length of stay in hospital) and mortality benefits in severe COPD exacerbations*

   Systemic glucocorticoids (1) *to reduce airway inflammation*

   Identify triggers for COPD exacerbation (1) *with chest radiography (pneumonia, pneumothorax) and ECG (acute coronary syndrome)*

   Urgent spirometry (0) *is contraindicated in situations of acute exacerbations of asthma or COPD*

   (max. 3 marks)

9. Yes (1) *as **smoking** is a risk factor for osteoporosis. So too are patients who have recurrent steroid prescriptions for their COPD.*

7.3

1. Delirium (1) *due to whatever organic cause, e.g. urinary tract infection, constipation, dehydration, hypoglycaemia, etc.*

   PLUS

   Dementia (1)

   Late-onset psychosis (1)

Stroke (1)

Brain tumour (1)

Charles Bonnet Syndrome (1) — visual hallucinations experienced by patients with significant visual impairment without other brain disease or psychiatric disorder, and who have insight that the perceptions are not real OR its cause, e.g. glaucoma, diabetic retinopathy, macular degeneration (0.5).

(max. 3 marks)

2. Onset of hallucinations (0.5) → acute onset denotes delirium (0.5)

   Accompanying auditory/tactile hallucinations (0.5) → suggest late-onset psychosis (0.5)

   Medication review (0.5) → certain drugs OR drug withdrawal (e.g. benzodiazepine) OR drug toxicity OR drug interactions can precipitate delirium (0.5)

   Alcohol history (0.5) → alcohol withdrawal (delirium tremens) can cause visual hallucinations (0.5)

   Localising symptoms (systemic review) (0.5) → for organic cause of delirium (0.5)

   Parkinsonian symptoms (e.g. resting tremor and limb stiffness) (0.5) → Parkinson disease may be associated with visual hallucinations (0.5)

   Cognitive history (0.5) → involvement of other cognitive domains against chronic onset may suggest dementia (0.5)

   (max. 4 marks)

3. Bedside cognitive test OR Abbreviated Mental Test OR Mini Mental State Examination (2)

   Visual acuity (1)

   Frontal lobe release signs (1)

   Gait (1)

   (max. 2 marks)

4. Diagnosis: Dementia (1)

   Aetiology: Dementia with Lewy bodies (1) OR Parkinson disease with dementia (1)

   (max. 2 marks)

5.	Limb ridigity (Parkinsonism) (1)

Postural hypotension (1) *due to antihypertensive medication, diabetic autonomic neuropathy and Parkinson disease.*

Visual impairment (1) *due to glaucoma or diabetic eye disease*

Hypoglycaemia (1) *due to diabetic medication or poor oral intake*

Cognitive impairment OR poor safety awareness (1) *due to dementia*

(max. 3 marks)

6.	Fall precautions (1)

Behavioural chart (1)

Capillary glucose monitoring (1)

Input-output charting (1)

Vital signs (0) *would routinely be done but not specifically for this patient's acute presentation*

(max. 2 marks)

7.	Cholinesterase inhibitor (1) *e.g. donepezil and rivastigmine.*

8.	Anticholinergics (1) can precipitate delirium in the elderly, especially those with dementia (1).

Antipsychotics (1) should be avoided in dementia with Lewy bodies due to neuroleptic sensitivity OR Parkinson disease dementia due to worsening of Parkinsonism (1).

(max. 2 marks)

7.4

1A.	Neuropathic (1)

Morphology of the ulcer: punched out (0.5), surrounded by callus (0.5)

Location of the ulcer: over pressure area (0.5)

Symptomatology of the ulcer: painless (0.5)

Granulating base (0)

1B. Hydrocolloid or hydrogel (1) *dressing is appropriate as it can provide some moisture to the wound bed and concurrent auto-lytic debridement as well.*

Any dressing with a topical antibiotic (0) — *indiscriminate use of antibiotics on non-infected wounds can cause the develop-ment of antibiotic resistance.*

Any foam or alginate dressing (0) — *these are for highly exu-dative wounds.*

1C. Minimise pressure (off-loading) (1)

Minimise friction and shear (1)

Maintain adequate nutrition (1) *(include ensuing good haemoglobin)*

(max. 2 marks)

2.   Catheter-associated urinary tract infection (1)

Infected foot ulcer (0)

3.   Right (0.5) renal (0.5) abscess (1)

4.   C (2) — *urine osmolality gives us an estimation of the action of antidiuretic hormones (ADHs), and that whether the patient is able to produce maximally concentrated urine in the pres-ence of hypernatraemia. The appropriate response in this set-ting is a high urine osmolality (>500 mOsm/kg). The plasma osmolality is expected to be high as the serum sodium is high, which is the main determinant of plasma osmolality.*

5.   A (2). *Water deficit = Total body water × (1-[140/serum sodium])*

Total body water = Body weight × 0.6

Hence water deficit = (70 × 0.6) × (1-[140/146]) = 2.1 L

6.   There is a defect in renal concentrating ability (1) *(diabetes insipidus)*

Failure to respond to vasopressin is more suggestive of nephro-genic diabetes insipidus. (1)

7.   Renal tubular damage due to gentamicin (1). *Other drugs that can cause nephrogenic diabetes insipidus are amphotericin B and lithium.*

Hypokalaemia (1), *if prolonged is associated with downregulation of aquaporin-2 water channel expression.*
(max. 1 mark)

8. D (2) — *presence of pyuria in an asymptomatic patient on an indwelling urinary catheter is NOT an indication for antimicrobial therapy.*

9. A (2) — *normal response: urine osmolality goes up after water deprivation due to the ADH effect to cause water retention resulting in maximally concentrated urine. B shows partial central diabetes insipidus (DI): there is usually some ADH secretion in response to water deprivation, which can be augmented after vasopressin administration. C shows primary polydipsia: in these patients, ADH secretion is normal, but they cannot produce maximally concentrated urine since the medullary concentration gradient is obliterated due to a large amount of water intake. D shows complete central DI: there is no response in terms of ADH secretion to water deprivation. The urine osmolality improves with vasopressin administration, but never reaches normal since the medullary concentration gradient is lost. E shows nephrogenic DI.*

7.5

1. Right breast lump (and nipple abnormality) (1)
    Hepatomegaly (1)
    Vertebral tenderness (1)
    Features of pleural effusion (1)
    Jaundice (1)
    Focal neurologic signs (1)
    (max. 4 marks)

2. B (2) — *a key principle of cancer management is staging an investigation to look for metastases to lungs, liver, bone and lymph nodes.*

3.   D (2) — *adjuvant therapy is meant to prevent recurrence; a close follow-up does not prevent recurrence. Treatment of estrogen-receptor positive breast cancer with hormonal therapy is effective and a good alternative to chemotherapy. Oestrogen in postmenopausal women comes mainly from adrenal glands, thus ovarian ablation, e.g. oophorectomy, ovarian irradiation or gonadotrophin-releasing hormone agonist, are useless.*

4.   C (2) — *hypercalcaemia can occur in patients with metastatic cancer, especially when there are bone metastases. Its presentation can be subtle!*

5.   Lower limb weakness OR gait unsteadiness (1)
     Lower limb sensory abnormalities, e.g. numbness, pins-and-needles sensation (1) — *usually ascending and reaches few levels below the actual level of cord compression.*
     Symptoms of bladder and/or bowel dysfunction, e.g. urinary retention (commonest) and incontinence (1) — *generally a late finding.*
     Any description of a clinical sign (0) — *question was specific for symptoms.*

6.   E (2)

7.   C (2) — *according to the European Society for Medical Oncology (ESMO) clinical practice guidelines, the opioid of first choice for moderate to severe cancer pain is oral morphine.*

8.   E (1) — *recommended first-line treatment as adjuvant analgesics for neuropathic cancer pain include gabapentin, pregabalin, nortriptyline and duloxetine.*

9.   Zoster (1) over the C8 dermatome (1)

Assessment Paper 8

8.1

1A. Intravenous (1) cefazolin (1) — *its spectrum of cover is narrower than amoxicillin/clavulanate.*

1B. Aztreonam (1) — *the cephalosporins are relatively contraindicated (though the risk of cross-reactivity is very low with third-generation ones). Amikacin is not an optimal drug as a sole agent for bacteraemia unless it is being combined with another antibiotic.*

2. 10–14 days (1)

3A. Central hypothyroidism (1)
Inappropriate thyroid stimulating hormone (TSH) for the low T4

3B. Pituitary damage secondary to previous cranial radiation (1)
Severe non-thyroidal illness (1)

4. The result, though within the laboratory normal range, cannot exclude hypoadrenalism (1) as the adrenal gland may still have sufficient reserve to maintain a "normal" cortisol level (1). *As yet, we do not know whether that reserve is sufficient enough to respond to an increased cortisol requirement of stress.*

5. Manifestations (or symptoms and signs) of hypocortisolism (1)
Manifestations (or symptoms and signs) of hypogonadism (1)
Manifestations (or symptoms and signs) of growth hormone deficiency (1)
Manifestations (or symptoms and signs) of hyperprolactinaemia (1)
Manifestations (or symptoms and signs) of mass effect (1), *e.g. headache and visual field abnormalities*
Manifestations (or symptoms and signs) of radiation effect (1), *e.g. visual field abnormalities and skin changes*

Recurrence of nasopharyngeal carcinoma (NPC) (1), *e.g. cranial nerve palsies and lymphadenopathy*

Manifestations (or symptoms and signs) of urinary tract abnormalities (1), *e.g. stone disease and prostatic enlargement*

Previous evaluation for diabetes mellitus (1)

Full drug history (1) — *some drugs can increase antidiuretic hormone (ADH) secretion or potentiate ADH action*

History of previous illness (1) *including treatment given* (max. 6 marks)

6.   Synacthen test (1) to rule out concomitant adrenal insufficiency as thyroxine replacement, before initiation of steroids can precipitate adrenal crisis (1).

7.   Stool for *Clostridium difficile* cytotoxin (1)

Stool for *Clostridium difficile* polymerase chain reaction (PCR) (0.5) *is not the choice of test as it is over-sensitive*

Stool culture (0.5) *takes more time and may result in a delay in diagnosis*

Stool microscopy (0)

(max. 1 mark)

8.   Oral (1) metronidazole OR vancomycin (1) *for 10–14 days*

Cessation of antibiotic (0) *is inappropriate here as he had bacteraemia, so the antibiotic must run its course*

8.2

1.   *An acute abdomen like this can have a very long list of differential diagnoses, but the MOST likely are (1 mark each):*
Perforated viscus (e.g. gastric/duodenal ulcer, colon or appendix)
Acute pancreatitis
Acute cholecystitis
Obstetric emergency (e.g. ruptured ectopic pregnancy)

Gynaecological emergency (e.g. ruptured ovarian cyst)

Severe ischaemic colitis (OR mesenteric ischaemia)

Leaking abdominal aortic aneurysm *(patients with ruptured aneurysm normally have high blood pressure and acute severe pain)*

Conditions with similar presentations usually without rebound and guarding are less likely (0 mark each): acute myocardial infarction, diabetic ketoacidosis *(pain from ileus due to acidosis and hypokalaemia),* ureteric colic, basal pulmonary embolism, acute intermittent porphyria, etc.

Intestinal obstruction (0) — *unlikely as she had no change in bowel habits or history of abdominal surgery to suggest adhesions*

(max. 4 marks)

2. Urine pregnancy test (1)

   Electrocardiogram (1)

   Chest X-ray (1)

   Serum ketones (1)

   Serum lipase (1)

   Cardiac enzymes (1)

   Lactate dehydrogenase (0.5) *as it is a marker of severity of acute pancreatitis*

   C-Reactive Protein (CRP) test (0.5) *as it is a marker of severity of acute pancreatitis*

   (max. 4 marks)

3. Eruptive xanthomas (0.5)

   Xanthelasma (0.5)

   Periumbilical ecchymosis (Cullen sign) (0.5)

   Flank ecchymosis (Grey Turner sign) (0.5)

   Lipemia retinalis (0.5)

   Jaundice (0.5)

   Tender shin nodules (pancreatitic panniculitis) (0.5)

   (max. 2 marks)

4. Acute pancreatitis (0.5) likely due to severe (0.5) hypertriglyc-
    eridemia (0.5), which is probably secondary to diabetes (0.5)
    and obesity (0.5).
    (max. 2 marks)
5. Recent binge alcohol consumption (1)
    History of biliary colic OR gallstone disease (1)
6. A No (0.5) — *low diagnostic yield in this setting*
    B Yes (0.5) — *as this patient has **severe** acute pancreatitis*
    C Yes (0.5)
    D No (0.5) — *she is haemodynamically unstable and currently
    has marked pain, nausea and vomiting*
    E No (0.5) — *not for all cases of acute pancreatitis unless
    clinically indicated*
    F Yes (0.5) — *when haemodynamically stable*
    G No (0.5) — *this patient is likely to have acute pancreatitis
    attributable to severe triglyceridaemia. If there is additional
    suspicion of gallstone disease or when loculated collections
    are suspected, only then should endoscopic retrograde cholan-
    giopancreatography (ERCP) be considered.*
    H Yes (0.5) — *in view of hyperglycaemia and possible concur-
    rent diabetic ketoacidosis in acute pancreatitis*
7. Necrosis of adipocytes OR "ghost cells" (1) — *due to lipolysis
    from pancreatic enzymes*
    Foamy macrophages (1) — *from ingested lipid*
    Calcium soap deposits (1) *in areas of fat necrosis (a form of
    dystrophic calcification)*
    Acute inflammation in **subcutaneous** layer (1) — *consistent
    with pancreatitic panniculitis*
    Vasculitic changes (0)
    (max. 2 marks)

8.3

1A. A cough persisting beyond two months is considered chronic and requires further evaluation (1).

1B. Haemoptysis occurring after exertion is more likely due to a sudden elevation in the left atrial pressure such as mitral stenosis (1).

1C. Nocturnal cough is suggestive of bronchial asthma (1)

2. Lung cancer (1)

Pulmonary tuberculosis (1)

Bronchiectasis (1)

Community-acquired pneumonia (0.5) — *would be highly unusual to cause such protracted symptoms (onset of community-acquired pneumonia is usually within days to short weeks).*

Chronic obstructive pulmonary disease (0.5) — *does not usually cause haemoptysis unless there is a co-existing second pathology, e.g. pulmonary tuberculosis or lung cancer.*

(max. 3 marks)

3A. Finger clubbing (0.5)

Hypertrophic pulmonary osteoarthropathy (0.5) — *see the expansion of the wrist joint*

Intrinsic muscle wasting (0.5) — *see the guttering on the dorsum of the hands*

(max. 1 mark)

3B. Miosis of right pupil (1)

Right hemifacial anhidrosis (1)

Right dilation lag (1) — *the miotic pupil takes a longer time to dilate when a bright light source is moved away from it*

Right enopthalmos (1) — *whether this is an actual or apparent phenomenon is still contentious*

Anisocoria (0.5) — *is not specific enough*

Muscle wasting (1) — *e.g. cheeks*

(max. 2 marks)

4. A (1) — *air entry appears to be completely compromised from the radiological evidence of the right upper lobemass.*
5. Mild tracheal deviation (1)
    Bony erosion of the right second rib (1)
    Elevated right hemidiaphragm (1)
    (max. 2 marks)
6. Tumour compression/invasion of the right recurrent laryngeal nerve (1) — *with vocal cord palsy*
    Chronic laryngitis due to chronic smoking (1)
    Vocal cord polyps due to chronic smoking (1)
    (max. 2 marks)
7. E → A → B → D → C (all answers must be correct to obtain 2 marks)
    As lung cancer is the most likely diagnosis, a pan-CT is important to further characterise the lung lesion and to stage the cancer. The next step is to plan for a biopsy to obtain tissue for histological diagnosis. Bronchoscopy or CT-guided lung biopsy would be appropriate. Sputum cytology has low sensitivity for the diagnosis of lung cancer and is thus ranked lower than a tissue biopsy. Pulmonary tuberculosis can mimic the presentation of lung cancer (upper lobe changes and haemoptysis) thus sputum for mycobacterial studies is a reasonable investigation in this scenario. Spirometry is contraindicated in patients with unexplained haemoptysis.
8. C (1) — *non-small cell lung carcinoma (NSCLC) is the most common primary lung cancer*
9. Lying down increases venous return and exacerbates the consequences of the superior vena cava obstruction (SVCO) (1).
10. B (2) — *the primary treatment for SVCO due to NSCLC includes treatment of the underlying cancer, which involves chemotherapy, radiotherapy or a combination of both. Life-threatening malignant SVCO may require endovascular stenting. The role of glucocorticoids is poorly studied in SVCO due to NSCLC but is believed to help reduce inflammation from the malignancy or radiotherapy that exacerbates SVCO.*

8.4

1. Acute or uncompensated (1) respiratory (0.5) acidosis (0.5)
   Hypoxaemia (0.5)
   (max. 2 marks)
2. Sinus tachycardia (1)
   Left ventricular hypertrophy (1): *S(V1) + R(V5) >35 mm*
3A. Asymmetrical (0.5) skin-coloured (1) knobbly or nodular (0.5)
   plaques (1)
   (max. 2 marks)
3B. Hyaluronic acid or glycosaminoglycan (1)
3C. Dorsum of feet (1)
   Sites of trauma (1)
   Less common sites, e.g. knees, shoulders, hands, fingers,
   elbows, arms and face (1)
   (max. 1 mark)
4. Fluid overload from cardiac failure (1)
5. Intravenous (1) diuretic (1)
   Any form of sodium replacement (0)
6. B, C and G (1 × 3 = 3 marks) — *as of the current time, the
   classes of medication that have been shown to reduce mortality
   rate in heart failure with* **reduced** *ejection fraction are beta-
   blockers, angiotensin system blockers (angiotensin converting
   enzyme (ACE) inhibitor or angiotensin-II blocker or angiotensin receptor-neprilysin inhibitor), mineralocorticoid receptor
   antagonists, hydralazine plus nitrate, and sodium-glucose co-
   transporter 2 inhibitors.*
7. Thyroid storm (1) — *the patient had fever, mental changes and
   cardiac involvement*
   Severe hypothyroidism (0.5) *per se very rarely causes fever
   and mental changes*
8. The risk of voice hoarseness from damage to recurrent laryngeal nerve (1) *is especially important as his occupation
   involves singing. An experienced head and neck surgeon would
   usually take precautions in preserving the laryngeal nerves.*

9. Hypocalcaemia (0.5) as the result of transient hypoparathyroidism (0.5) due to manipulation of the blood supply to or removal of the parathyroid glands during surgery (1).

10. Trousseau sign (1): *inflate the sphygmomanometer to 20 mmHg above the systolic blood pressure for 3–5 minutes, watch for abnormal movement of the hand and wrist.*
    Chvostek sign (1): *tapping the facial nerve (2 cm anterior to external auditory meatus) will result in the contraction of the ipsilateral facial muscles.*

8.5

1. E and F (1 × 2 = 2 marks) — *the patient with Addison's disease is more often dehydrated rather than fluid overloaded. Given her longstanding history and the mentioned absence of other symptoms, constrictive pericarditis cannot be a cause of such longstanding swelling. Lymphoedema (due to pelvic malignancy, for instance) does not improve with diuretics; over a few years, the pelvic malignancy should have manifested itself, and the lymphedema is likely to become chronic with skin hardening. The longstanding duration of symptoms also makes rapidly progressive glomerulonephritis (GN) an unlikely cause, although GN can give both hypertension and oedema. Rheumatoid arthritis can give swelling from either the effusion itself at the ankle joints or synovial thickening. Systemic lupus may be associated commonly with nephrotic syndrome.*

2A. May imply idiopathic cyclic oedema (in women) (1)

2B. May suggest a loss of protein from the gut (either from malabsorption or a protein-losing gastroenteropathy) (1)

3. C and F (1 × 2 = 2 marks) — *a useful history to obtain from the patient with lower limb swelling is the onset or aggravation of symptoms with the introduction of medication.*

4A. Her total protein is markedly elevated (1). The relatively low albumin suggests that the contribution to it is likely from a high amount of globulins (1). *Hyperglobulinaemia can occur in acute infections, dehydration, paraproteinaemias like multiple myeloma, and autoimmune diseases like lupus and lymphomas.*

4B. Paraproteinaemia or multiple myeloma (1). It is based on a constellation of findings in an older (0.5) lady with generalised aches (0.5), anaemia (0.5), markedly elevated erythrocyte sedimentation rate (ESR) (0.5), elevated total protein (and likely globulin) (0.5) and mild renal impairment (0.5).

5. Serum protein electrophoresis (1) *can be used to identify the different proteins present based on their molecular properties. They help to identify any characteristic band patterns seen in different types of paraproteinemia. Monoclonal bands may be seen in multiple myeloma, Waldenstrom's or monoclonal gammopathy of uncertain significance (MGUS). Polyclonal bands may be seen in connective tissue diseases such as systemic lupus erythematosus (SLE), autoimmune hepatitis and infections, and other inflammatory states.*
Urine protein electrophoresis (0.5)
Calcium studies (1) *are important as hypercalcaemia can occur commonly in about a quarter of patients with multiple myeloma due to bone demineralisation. Hypercalcaemia may also have a prognostic significance.*
Skeletal survey (0) *is not appropriate at this stage*
Bone marrow examination (0) *is not appropriate at this stage*
(max. 2 marks)

6A. The albumin-creatinine ratio measures small amounts of albumin in the urine (microalbuminuria). It does not measure the low molecular-sized light chains (1).

6B. Light chains can precipitate in renal tubules and cause tubular damage (myeloma kidney) (1)

Light chains may cause glomerulosclerosis (1)

Light chains may be associated with amyloid nephropathy (1)

The presence of light chains may promote the aggravation of renal disease when radiocontrast media are used for imaging studies (1).

(max. 2 marks)

7A. Bone marrow biopsy (aspiration and trephine) (1)

7B. Plasma cells may be increased to 10% or more in multiple myeloma (1) — *2–3% in normal individuals.*

Plasma cells may be abnormal (0.5), *e.g. multinucleate*

(max. 1 mark)

8. This X-ray shows the classic changes of multiple myeloma: distinct, well-defined and punched-out lucent lesions (without surrounding reactive changes, unlike what is seen in secondaries) (1). *Some have mistakenly labelled it as "pepper pot skull", which is a more granular appearing skull typical of severe hyperparathyroidism.*

Assessment Paper 9

9.1

1. A (2) — *Osteoporosis is defined using densitometric criteria of the lowest T-score of the spine, total hip or femoral neck or forearm of <–2.5. However, T-scores should not be used when interpreting bone mineral density (BMD) in* **premenopausal** *women. The International Society for Clinical Densitometry (ISCD) recommends the use of BMD Z-scores (comparison to age-matched norms) rather than T-scores (comparison to premenopausal norms) at the lumbar spine, hip and forearm. A Z-score ≤ –2.0 should be interpreted as "below the expected range for age" and a Z-score > –2.0 as "within the expected*

range for age". The diagnostic categories of "osteopenia" and "osteoporosis" based solely upon the BMD T-score should not be applied in premenopausal women.

2. A review of her medication for steroids (oral, intramuscular, intra articular, inhaled, intranasal and topical) as well as supplements and traditional medication that may be adulterated with corticosteroids (1).

3. Easy bruising (1)

    Facial plethora (1)

    Proximal muscle weakness (1)

    Purplish striae (1)

    Fine thin skin (1)

    One must have a high index of suspicion for Cushing's syndrome in this premenopausal lady with unexplained low BMD, hypertension and marked unexplained weight gain. While the spectrum of clinical presentation is very broad in Cushing's syndrome, the aforementioned features are more discriminatory.

    Dorsocervical hump (0.5)

    Supraclavicular fullness (0.5)

    Acne (0.5)

    These other features (as well as hirsutism, facial fullness) are common in the general population and are less discriminatory

    (max. 3 marks)

4A. Adrenocorticotropic hormone (ACTH) independent OR Adrenal (1) Cushing's syndrome (1) — *this patient has a non-suppressed 1 mg dexamethasone test and low ACTH, which reflect the negative feedback suppression of pituitary corticotrophs by excess cortisol. We also have to bear in mind that the overnight dexamethasone may have a 5% false positive rate, although, in this patient, the context does not suggest so.*

4B. Both the 24-hour urinary free cortisol (UFC) were within normal limits with normal urinary volumes. This happens particularly in **subclinical** Cushing's syndrome (1) — *the 24-hour UFC is the most sensitive test in the evaluation of Cushing's syndrome.*

5. Right (1) adrenal gland (1)

6. Unilateral OR Right (0.5) adrenalectomy (0.5)

7. I (1) — *a fine-needle biopsy is not needed to exclude malignancy prior to adrenalectomy in this patient. It is associated with the risk of bleeding and is unnecessary prior to adrenalectomy.*

A (1) — *diabetes mellitus is a complication of Cushing's syndrome and screening for diabetes, and if present, optimisation of glycemic control will improve the perioperative outcome.*

A (1) — *adrenal insufficiency occurs in about half of patients undergoing adrenalectomy for subclinical hypercortisolism. Perioperative intravenous steroid cover until the recovery of the hypothalamus-pituitary axis is necessary.*

8. Hypokalemia with **inappropriate** kaliuresis [24-hr urine K > 20 mmol/L] (1)

The renal potassium loss cannot be attributed to hypomagnaesium or hypocalcaemia (1), *as both may induce hypokalaemia by increasing distal potassium secretion, and both may also indicate renal tubular dysfunction.*

Metabolic alkalosis (1) *as indicated by elevated serum bicarbonate*

The presence of metabolic alkalosis, hypokalaemia and hypertension is suspicious for either mineralocorticoid excess or increased activation of the mineralocorticoid receptor (1).

(max. 3 marks)

9. The mineralocorticoid receptor has the **same affinity** for aldosterone and cortisol (0.5). However, it is physiologically protected from cortisol by the activity of **11β-hydroxysteroid**

dehydrogenase type 2 enzyme, which inactivates cortisol to cortisone (0.5).

In Cushing's syndrome, the **excess cortisol overwhelms the 11β-hydroxysteroid dehydrogenase type 2 enzyme** (0.5), leading to the activation of the mineralocorticoid receptor, producing the **apparent mineralocorticoid effects** (0.5) *such as hypokalaemia, metabolic alkalosis and hypertension.*

9.2

1A. Dysphagia (1)
   Constipation (1)
   Poor oral health (poor dentition, oral ulcers, xerostomia) (1)
   (max. 2 marks)
1B. Delirium (1)
   Depression (1)
   Pain (OA flare) (1)
   Iatrogenesis/medication side-effects (1)
   Malignancy (1)
   (max. 2 marks)
2. Capillary blood glucose (1)
3. Atrial fibrillation (1)
   Downsloping ST-T depression ("reverse tick") in lateral leads (1)
   Right axis deviation (1)
   (max. 2 marks)
4. Digoxin toxicity (2)
5. Discontinuation of all oral medication (1) — *this patient has the perfect scenario for digoxin toxicity — renal impairment, hypokalaemia and a fairly high dose of digoxin for an 80-year-old. Digoxin and potassium compete for the same receptors. Enalapril can also accentuate digoxin toxicity. Other medications should be suspended as the patient is drowsy and will be*

prone to aspiration. Risperidone is sedating, and she is at risk of hypoglycaemia due to poor intake.

> **PLUS**
> Judious intravenous potassium replacement (1)
> Intravenous hydration (1)
> Empirical intravenous amoxicillin-clavulante (0.5) for pneumonia, after obtaining blood cultures (0.5)
> Intravenous sodium correction (0)
> Any antiarrhythmic treatment (0)
> (max. 2 marks)

6. Oropharyngeal dysphagia (1)
7. Alzheimer's dementia (1)
    Drug-induced parkinsonism secondary to risperidone (1)
    Parkinson disease (0.5)
    (max. 2 marks)
8. Alendronate-induced oesophagitis (2)
9. A, B and C ($1 \times 3 = 3$ marks)

9.3

1A. Fourth (4th) cranial nerve palsy (1) — *this is a compensatory mechanism to overcome the extorsion deficit of the abnormal eye.*

1B. Sixth (6th) cranial nerve (1) — *this is a compensatory mechanism to overcome the action of the weak lateral rectus.*

2A. Myasthenia Gravis (1)
    Hypoglycaemia (1)
    Adverse drug reaction, e.g. sildenafil and pregabalin (1)
    (max. 1 mark)

2B. Guillain Barre syndrome (or variants) (1)
    Brain stem stroke (1)
    (max. 1 mark)

2C. Weber syndrome (midbrain stroke) (1)

3A. Horner syndrome (1)

3B. Third (3rd) cranial nerve palsy (1)

3C. Horner syndrome (1) — *in Horner syndrome, the Müller's muscle is weak because of the sympathetic innervation, but the levator palpebrae muscle supplied by the 3rd nerve can overcome it.*

4. Left 3rd cranial nerve palsy (1) as there is near complete (0.5) ptosis and the left eye is down and out (0.5) (*a divergent gaze*)

5A. Extrinsic compressive lesion (1) — *where the parasympathetic fibers, which run on the outer surface of the 3rd nerve (pia matter) being affected, thus pupillary constrictive reactions are compromised.*

5B. Parasympathetic fibers are spared, and as such, it can suggest a more central lesion (vasa nervorum) within the 3rd nerve fibers (1), *e.g. vasculitis, diabetes mellitus mononeuropathy.*

6. The patient has both 3rd and 6th nerve palsies (2) — *it would be hard to tell from these pictures if he had complete ophthalmoplegia. The actual patient had complete ophthalmoplegia of the left eye.*

7A. Cavernous sinus thrombosis (1)
Superior orbital fissure syndrome (1)
(max. 1 mark)

7B. Nasopharyngeal carcinoma (1)
Radiation therapy (1)
Leukaemia or lymphoma (1)
(max. 1 mark)

8. Asymmetrical (1) extended (1) bitemporal hemianopia (1) — *strongly suggesting a chiasmal compressive lesion either arising from or infiltrating the pituitary gland at the chiasma.*
(max. 2 marks)

9. *The combination of bitemporal hemianopia with the 3rd and 6th cranial nerve involvement would suggest an infiltrative process*

*that involves **both** the pituitary and the cavernous sinus.* This could represent a highly invasive pituitary tumour *(seen some-times in aggressive prolactinomas, rarely in malignant tumours)* or in metastases — *this patient had an aggressive invasive pitui-tary tumour.* (2)

9.4

1. Sallow and/or hyperpigmented appearance (1)
    Excoriations (1) *due to pruritus*
    Uraemic frost (1) — *urea secreted by eccrine glands giving an appearance of salt crystals; a rare phenomenon seen in very severe uraemic patients.*
    (max. 2 marks)

2A. **The presence of HBC total antibody in the absence of HBsAg and anti-HBs** can occur due to anti-HBs falling to undetectable levels after recovery from acute Hepatitis B (1) or in the setting of chronic hepatitis, where the HBsAg titre has fallen below the cut-off for detection (1). *This phenomenon can be present in 10–20% of the population in endemic countries.* It can reflect occult Hepatitis B infection (1)
    Sometimes, an isolated positive HBC total antibody result may be due to false positivity (1).
    (max. 3 marks)
    Additional notes to clarify the concept: HBsAg is the serologi-cal hallmark of HBV infection. If the patient is HBsAg negative and anti-HBs positive, the patient is immune to Hepatitis B. In this setting, HBC total antibody helps to differentiate between immunity from vaccination (HBC total antibody negative) as opposed to a previous infection (HBC total antibody positive).

2B. An HBV DNA assay (1) *is recommended to exclude viraemia. Note that even if anti-HBs are positive and the patient is immune, some experts recommend an HBV DNA assay if the patient is HBC total antibody positive, even though the chance of transmission from such patients is very small.*

3. C (1) — *cather-related bloodstream infections (CRBSIs) are a recognised complication of haemodialysis catheters. If there is no other obvious source of infection in a patient on a dialysis catheter, a CRBSI should be suspected. The greatest predictors of infective mortality in dialysis accesses are, in ascending order: arteriovenous fistulas (AVFs), arteriovenous grafts (AVGs), cuffed dialysis catheters, and uncuffed catheters.*

4. Paired blood cultures drawn from the catheter and a peripheral vein (1)

   Blood cultures (0.5)

   Removal of catheter and sending tip for culture (0)

   (max. 1 mark)

5. ***Staphylococcus aureus*** (1), *followed by Staphylococcus epidermides (0), form the bulk of infections and accounts for nearly 50% of CRBSI. Other common organisms include gram-negative bacteria (Escherichia coli, Pseudomonas species, Klebsiella species) and enterococci. Methicillin-resistant Staphylococcus aureus (MRSA) bacteraemia was 100 times more common in dialysis patients than the general population according to a study, and this was compounded 8–10 times in patients dialysing via catheters versus AVFs.*

6. B (2) — *catheter removal and systemic antibiotics are the treatment of choice in the setting of CRBSI with methicillin-sensitive Staphylococcus aureus (MSSA) and MRSA. Even Pseudomonas and fungal CRBSI necessitate catheter removal. Catheter salvage and systemic antibiotics with an antibiotic line lock can be considered in infections with Staph epidermides and gram-negative organisms except for Pseudomonas. Irrespective of the organism, if the patient is haemodynamically unstable or if he remains febrile or bacteraemic after 48–72 hours of appropriate antibiotics, the catheter must be removed.*

7.   C (1) — *the dialysis catheter should only be inserted when repeat blood cultures are negative.*

8.   Resistance to vancomycin (1) — *some MRSA strains exhibit resistance to vancomycin, and guidelines recommend that agents other than vancomycin be considered when the minimum inhibitory concentration (MIC) is 2 microgram/ml or more.*
    Inadequate dosing with sub-therapeutic trough levels (1) — *a vancomycin trough level of 15–20 mg/L is warranted in bacteraemia and deep-seated infection with MRSA, but a level of 10–15 is considered adequate for non-severe infections such as soft tissue infections.*
    Metastatic seeding of infection (1) — *these sites can include heart valve (infective endocarditis), lungs (septic emboli, lung abscess, empyema), central nervous system (brain abscess, meningitis), abdomen (liver abscess, splenic abscess) and musculoskeletal (discitis, osteomyelitis, septic arthritis).*
    Fungaemia (0.5)
    Drug fever (0)
    (max. 3 marks)

9.   Drug-induced (1) — *drug-induced immune thrombocytopenia (DITP) is the most common mechanism, and vancomycin is a well-known cause of drug-induced thrombocytopenia.*
    Disseminated intravascular coagulation (1)
    Heparin-induced thrombocytopenia (HIT) (0.5) — *HIT is not uncommon in haemodialysis patients. HIT is due to drug-dependent antibodies that also activate platelets and are associated with venous and arterial thrombosis. The 4Ts score, which is used to estimate the clinical probability of HIT, takes into account the degree and timing of thrombocytopenia, the presence of thrombosis and the presence of other causes of thrombocytopenia. In this clinical setting, ongoing sepsis features suggestive of disseminated intravascular coagulation, the*

absence of thrombosis and the fact that the patient has been on heparin on dialysis for a few weeks before he developed thrombocytopenia make HIT a less likely etiology, and it is more likely to be due to severe sepsis and disseminated intravascular coagulation.

(max. 2 marks)

10. Mitral valve vegetations (infective endocarditis) (1)
    Flow murmur (1)
11. Trans-oesophageal echocardiography (1)

9.5

1. History of painful eye with impaired vision (1) — *uveitis?*
   History of painful swelling of a digit (1) — *dactylitis?*
   History of scaly rash on scalp/limbs/body (1) — *psoriasis?*
   History of recurrent bloody diarrhoea (1) — *inflammatory bowel disease?*
   Good response to nonsteroidal anti-inflammatory drugs (NSAIDs) (1)
   Family history for spondyloarthritis (SpA) (1)
   Any associated constitutional symptoms such as fatigue or weight loss (0.5)
   Radiation of pain down the leg (0.5) — *sciatica usually refers to disc disease, which is unlikely based on a history of the inflammatory nature of the pain.*
   Onset/tempo/recurrence/degree of severity/nature/aggravating factors of the pain (0) *are good questions in history-taking but not diagnostic enough for this specific question.*
   (max. 4 marks)
2. Schober's (or Modified Schober's) test (1)
3. XR of the sacroiliac joints (1) to *look for evidence of sacroiliitis*

MRI of the sacroiliac joints (1) *can detect active inflammation in the sacroiliac joints and spine that is not visible on plain radiography. Sacroiliitis can be detected by an MRI years before radiographic sacroiliitis is apparent.*

HLA-B27 (1) *is useful as part of the clinical assessment. It is the primary disease susceptibility gene for ankylosing spondylitis. It is by no means a screening test and should be used appropriately and interpreted in the clinical context.*

Inflammatory markers: C-reactive protein (CRP) (1) and/or Erythrocyte Sedimentation Rate (ESR) (0.5)

Ultrasound heel (0.5) *can confirm and/or quantify the extent of the plantar fasciitis (which is a form of enthesitis).*

Any left shoulder and right knee investigation (0)

(max. 3 marks)

4A. I (1) — *in general, rest is bad for patients with low back pain. In patients with inflammatory low back pain, exercise relieves rather than aggravates the pain.*

4B. I (1) — *the heel pain is causing only minor clinical symptoms so treatment modalities other than an injection would be more appropriate initially.*

4C. A (1)

4D. A (1) — *physiotherapy is one of the most widely used forms of treatment adopted for gaining relief from low back pain. Physical therapy can also help improve posture and range of motion for patients with ankylosing spondylitis.*

5A. Atrial (P waves) and ventricular (QRS complexes) activities are independent of each other (1)

Ventricular rate ~50 bpm (0.5)

Atrial rate ~100 bpm (0.5)

5B. Third-degree OR Complete heart block (1)

6. Association with ankylosing spondylitis (1) *and other rheumatic diseases*

Acute (viral) myocarditis (1)

7. B (1) — *IV atropine (0.5 mg) stat should be administered while awaiting transcutaneous pacing. May repeat to a total dose of 3 mg.*
8. Implantable pacemaker (1)
   Aortic valve replacement (0) *is indicated in symptomatic patients with severe aortic valve regurgitation.*
9. Aortic valve insufficiency/regurgitation (1) *due to thickening and displacement of aortic valve cusps and dilatation of aortic root*
   Mitral valve abnormality (0) *less likely*
   Left ventricular hypertrophy or cardiomegaly (0) *are secondary changes not primary.*

Assessment Paper 10

10.1

1. Severe shock (1)
   Acute meningitis (1)
   Septic or sepsis associated encephalopathy (1)
   (max. 2 marks)
2. B (2) — *standard protocol for severely hypoglycaemic patients who are unable to take it orally. IM glucagon should be considered if unable to obtain intravenous access.*
3. Aggressive fluid resuscitation (1)
   Empirical broad-spectrum parenteral antibiotics (0.5) after septic workup (0.5)
   Transfer to intensive care (0) — *premature at this stage while outcome of initial stablisation is yet unknown.*
4. B (2) — *standard protocol to repeat the hypoglycaemia rescue as above if unresponsive within 15–30 minutes after initial treatment.*

5A. Severe (0.5) high anion-gap (1) metabolic acidosis (0.5)
Renal failure or impairment (0) — *not the most significant one because it is not as life-threatening as the severe acidosis!*

5B. Lactic acidosis (1) *from shock and possibly contributed by metformin too*
Renal failure (1)
Drugs/toxins (1), *e.g. salicylate, methanol, ethylene glucol, isopropyl alcohol*
Diabetic ketoacidosis (0)
(max. 2 marks)

5C. Continue aggressive hydration (1)
Treat underlying causes of hypotension (1)
Intravenous sodium bicarbonate (1) replacement
Oral sodium bicarbonate (0) replacement
Consider dialysis if acidosis is refractory (1)
(max. 3 marks)

6. A (2) — *sulphonyurea is the most likely to cause hypoglycaemia*

7. Acquired perforating dermatosis (1) — *monomorphic crateriform circular erythematous nodules*
Prurigo nodularis (1)
Eczema (0.5) — *a rather vague term for such morphologically distinct lesions*
Diabetic dermopathy (0)
Scabies (0)
Folliculitis (0)
(max. 2 marks)

8. A (1) — *a potent topical corticosteroid ointment is most suitable as first-line treatment. If that fails, one can consider intralesional corticosteroid.*

10.2

1A. Inflammatory bowel disease (1)

Crohn's disease (1) *is the more likely condition though it still needs to be proven*

Ulcerative colitis (0.5) *very uncommonly has oral ulceration*

Chronic malabsorption (0.5) *is a consequence of the above underlying condition*

(max. 1 mark)

1B. Human Immunodeficiency virus (HIV) infection (1)

PLUS many differentials but these are the most important:

Cytomegalovirus colitis (1)

Tuberculous colitis (1)

(max. 1 mark)

2A. Clubbing (1)

Koilonychia (1)

Beau's lines (1)

Pitting (0.5) *in psoriasis, which may be associated with Crohn's disease*

(max. 2 marks)

2B. Blood on glove (1)

Anal/rectal stricture and/or fissure (1)

Perianal fistula and/or abscess (1)

Perianal skin tags (1)

Haemorrhoids (1)

(max. 2 marks)

3. Dilated colon (1)

Faecal loading (1)

Loss of colonic shadow in his left lower abdomen (1)

(max. 2 marks)

4. Stool calprotectin (1)

Stool PCR infection panel (1)

Stool tuberculosis PCR (1)
Stool for microscopy for parasites (1)
Stool occult blood test (1)
(max. 3 marks)
5. Stricture (1)
    Ulceration (1)
    Mucosal inflammation (1)
    Cobble stone appearance (1)
    (max. 2 marks)
6. F, G and H (1 × 3 = 3 marks) — *other differentials include Behcet's disease, tuberculosis, Crohn's disease, cytomegalovirus colitis.*
7. Myelotoxicity from azathioprine (0.5) due to deficiency in thiopurine methyltransferase activity (0.5)
    Drug interaction (0.5), which potentiates the action of azathioprine (0.5), *e.g. allopurinol*
    Idiosyncratic (0.5) marrow suppression due to methotrexate (0.5) — *dose-dependent marrow suppression usually occurs at higher doses, which are unlikely to be prescribed at the outset of the disease.*
    Megaloblastic anaemia due to B12 malabsorption in the terminal ileum (0.5) *is plausible but unlikely as active treatment had commenced, and the counts do not plummet so acutely.*
    (max. 2 marks)
8. Granulocyte colony-stimulating factor (1)
    Folinic acid (0.5) — *useful only in methotrexate toxicity*
    (max. 1 mark)

10.3

1. Did she bite her tongue during the seizure? (1)
    How fast did she regain consciousness? (1) *It is gradual after a seizure whereas it is prompt after a faint.*

Was she confused and/or drowsy upon regaining consciousness? (1)

Did she notice bowel and/or urinary incontinence? (1)

(max. 2 marks)

2. Any chronic alcohol intake or withdrawal? (1)

Any use of recreational drugs? (1)

Any sleep deprivation? (1)

Note that an intake of oestrogen-containing oral contraceptives can also cause seizures.

(max. 2 marks)

3. Electrolytes including serum calcium, magnesium, phosphate (max. 1 mark)

Serum glucose (1)

Blood or urine toxicology (1)

An electrocardiogram (ECG) (1) *as cardiogenic syncope due to an arrhythmia can be complicated by a secondary hypoxic seizure*

CT brain scan (1)

Chest X-ray (1) — *especially if aspiration after a seizure is suspected on clinical grounds.*

An electroencephalogram (EEG) (0.5) — *while the presence of epileptiform abnormalities predicts an increased risk for seizure recurrence after a first unprovoked seizure, note that a normal EEG does not rule out epilepsy.*

(max. 3 marks)

4. Drowsiness (1)

Giddiness (1)

Weight gain (1)

Tremor (1)

Nausea or Vomiting (1)

Easy bruising (1) — *secondary to thrombocytopenia*

Teratogenicity (1) — *hence give only if she is certain she does not intend to conceive!*

(max. 2 marks)

5. For unprovoked seizures *(whether single or recurrent),* she should stop driving (1). Driving can resume after a seizure-free period of at least 10 years (0.5) with a normal EEG (0.5), no structural brain lesion (0.5), normal neurological examination (0.5) and if the patient is not on any anti-epileptic drugs (0.5) — *see Singapore Medical Association guidelines, 2011.* (max. 2 marks)

    Generally, for a provoked seizure, driving can resume after a seizure-free period of at least one year with a normal EEG.

6. Check adherence/compliance to therapy (1)

    Check for drug interactions, especially drugs that increase the clearance of valproate (1), *e.g. rifampicin.*

    Look for a provoking/triggering factor (1), *e.g. infection, stroke.*

    (max. 2 marks)

7A. Tuberculoma (1)

    Cryptococcoma (1)

    Aspergilloma (1)

    Neurocysticercosis (1) — caused by an infection with *Taenia solium. It is endemic in many regions of Central and South America, sub-Saharan Africa, India and Asia, and is associated with tight clustering in households and poor sanitisation.*
    Cerebral toxoplasmosis (1) — this infection has a worldwide distribution and is caused by the intracellular protozoan parasite, *Toxoplasma gondii.* It usually affects AIDS patients without appropriate prophylaxis.

    Cerebral abscess

    (max. 2 marks)

7B. Cerebral metastasis (1)

    Glioma (1)

    Neurosarcoidosis (1)

    (max. 2 marks)

8. Rifampicin + isoniazid + ethambutol + levofloxacin + pyrazinamide (0.5 each but max. 2 marks)
   Pyridoxine (0.5)
   Dexamethasone (0.5)
   (max. 3 marks)

10.4

1. Weakness of arms (1)
   Numbness of arms (1)
   Painful joints of upper limbs (1)
   Slippery surface on ladder (1)
   (max. 2 marks)
2. Osteopenia (1) *within thinned cortices*
   Supracondylar (0.5) pathological fracture (1)
   Osteoporosis (0.5) — *one cannot diagnose osteoporosis from simple radiology*
   (max. 2 marks)
3. D and E (1 × 2 = 2 marks) — *most fractures in osteogenesis imperfecta occur before puberty (he was previously well), although milder varieties may present in adulthood. Multiple myeloma occurs most commonly in those who are aged above 60 years. Cushing's syndrome (exogenous or endogenous), hypogonadism and hyperparathyroidism may be responsible for secondary osteoporosis and should be suspected, particularly in the young male presenting with a low impact fracture.*
4. D and E (1 × 2 = 2 marks) — *primary polydipsia describes a habitual tendency to drink water and should not be associated with other comorbidities like body aches and pains; it certainly is not associated with a pathological fracture. Thyrotoxicosis presenting with polyuria and polydipsia is uncommon in humans, although it is a common feature in feline presentations.*

5.   D and E ($1 \times 2 = 2$ marks) — *the man has no clinical features to suggest Cushing's syndrome or hypogonadism. His acute presentation of fractures (which requires intervention) together with the dehydrated status necessitates urea, creatinine and electrolytes measurements. The combination of polyuria and polydipsia in a patient with osteoporosis and a pathological fracture warrants exclusion of hypercalcaemia, particularly if an intervention for the fracture is planned. Calcium measurements should preferably be done with simultaneous phosphate measurements and albumin for a determination of the corrected calcium, should the albumin be grossly abnormal.*

6A. A simultaneous low serum phosphate generally suggests that the hypercalcaemia is driven by parathyroid hormone (PTH) or PTH-related peptide (1) *as they have a phosphaturic effect.*

6B. An overdose of Vitamin D can cause severe hypercalacaemia (1). *As such, a history of exogenous Vitamin D ingestion should be sought for in anyone with hypercalcaemia.*

6C. Urinary calcium can help differentiate hyperparathyroidism (urinary calcium increased) from familial **hypocalciuric** hypercalcaemia (1).

7.   "Hungry Bone Syndrome" — continual high bone turnover due to the very high parathyroid hormone prior to surgery (1). After a dramatic drop in the parathyroid hormone, the rate of skeletal mineralisation exceeds the rate of osteoclast-mediated bone resorption, resulting in hypocalcaemia.

8.   Urgent (0.5) intravenous (1) calcium (1) *administration to overcome the cramps and normalise the calcium levels* (max. 2 marks)

9.   *The X-ray shows the classic radiological changes of primary hyperparathyroidism:*
Resorption of the terminal phalanx (1)
Subperiosteal bone resorption (1), *particularly on the radial aspects of the middle phalanges.*

10. On careful review of the original X-ray, two oval-shaped translucencies are noted in the shaft of the humerus arising from the intramedullary cavities (1). These are "brown tumours" (1) — this is a bone lesion that arises in the setting of excess osteoclast activity.

    The mandible X-ray shows a similar appearance in this patient. These "brown tumours" are most commonly found in the maxilla or mandible, although any bone may be affected. This young man had a supracondylar fracture that involved the brown tumour site.

10.5

1. Presence of frothy urine (1)
   Decrease in urine volume (1)
   Any discolouration in urine OR gross hematuria (1)
   (max. 2 marks)
2. Many sexually-transmitted infections are associated with nephrotic syndrome, *e.g. Hepatitis B and Hepatitis C (membranous and membranoproliferative glomerulonephritis), syphilis (membranous glomerulonephritis) and HIV (focal segmental glomerulosclerosis).* (2)
3. Elevated jugular venous pressure together with a sharp "y" (and/or "x") descent is suggestive of constrictive pericarditis, *an important consideration in a patient with peripheral oedema, and ascites without orthopnoea!* (2)
4. Duplex ultrasound (1) of renal veins to look for renal vein thrombosis (1)
5. Nephrotic syndrome (1) due to minimal change disease (1)
6A. Oral (1) prednisolone (1)
6B. Diuretic (1) *for symptomatic relief*
    Fluid restriction (1)
    A low-salt diet (0.5)

Intravenous albumin (0.5) — *usually combined with intravenous frusemide in massive anasarca or significant respiratory distress*

Anti-lipid agents (0.5) — *may be considered if the lipid panel does not improve with the primary treatment of the nephrotic syndrome (which likely caused the hyperlipidaemia)*

Anticoagulation (0.5) — *for primary prevention (though controversial)*

Corticosteroid-sparing agents (0) — *e.g. cyclosphosphamide, ciclosporin are used in steroid-resistant cases*

(max. 2 marks)

7.   Pulmonary thromboembolism (1)
Pulmonary congestion (1)
Chest infection (1)
(max. 2 marks)

8.   An electrocardiogram (ECG) (1)
    PLUS
    Chest X-ray (1)
    Arterial blood gas (1)
    D-dimer (1)
    Cardiac enzymes (0.5)
    CT pulmonary artery (0) *is not the immediate investigation*
    NT-proBNP (0)
    (max. 1 mark)

9.   Oxygen supplementation (1) *by nasal prongs or face mark till oxygen saturation goes above 95%*
Inform doctor stat if oxygen saturation falls below 95% (1)
Hourly parameters (0.5)
Continuous pulse oximetry (0.5)
(max. 2 marks)

CPSIA information can be obtained
at www.ICGtesting.com
Printed in the USA
FSHW021815010521
80889FS